I ♥ Orgasms

A GUIDE TO MORE

SECOND EDITION

DORIAN SOLOT & MARSHALL MILLER

WITH MAYBE BURKE

hachette
BOOKS

New York

Copyright © 2022 by Dorian Solot and Marshall Miller
Illustrations © 2007 by Shirley Chiang
"Absolut Impotence." Reprinted by permission of Adbusters Media Foundation
Vulva anatomy illustration. © Cary Bell. Courtesy of Cary Bell

Cover design by Terri Sirma
Cover copyright © 2022 by Hachette Book Group, Inc.

Hachette Go, an imprint of Hachette Books
Hachette Book Group
1290 Avenue of the Americas
New York, NY 10104
HachetteGo.com
Facebook.com/HachetteGo
Instagram.com/HachetteGo

Second Edition: December 2022

Hachette Books is a division of Hachette Book Group, Inc.

The Hachette Go and Hachette Books name and logos are trademarks of Hachette Book Group, Inc.

The publisher is not responsible for websites (or their content) that are not owned by the publisher.

Library of Congress Cataloging-in-Publication Data

Names: Solot, Dorian, author. | Miller, Marshall, 1974– author. | Burke, Maybe, author.
Title: I love orgasms : a guide to more / Dorian Solot and Marshall Miller with Maybe Burke.
Other titles: I [heart] female orgasm
Description: Second edition. | New York : Hachette Go, [2022] | Includes index.
Identifiers: LCCN 2022027623 | ISBN 9780306874970 (paperback) | ISBN 9780306874963 (ebook)
Subjects: LCSH: Orgasm. | Masturbation. | Sex instruction. | Female orgasm. | Female masturbation.
Classification: LCC HQ31 .S666 2022 | DDC 613.9/6—dc23/eng/20220819
LC record available at https://lccn.loc.gov/2022027623

ISBNs: 978-0-306-87497-0 (trade paperback); 978-0-306-87496-3 (ebook)

Printed in the United States of America

LSC-C

Printing 1, 2022

contents

Orgasms:
What's Not to Love?

Sexual pleasure is a human right that encompasses the freedom
of expression—free from judgement, coercion, and stigma.
—Dr. Tlaleng Mofokeng, South African physician and
United Nations Special Rapporteur on the Right to Health

For some, standing on a stage in front of a packed auditorium, talking
about vulvas, penises, and orgasms would be a scene from a sweat-soaked, heart-
pounding nightmare. For us, it's just another day at work. As independent sex
educators, we've spent the last two decades traveling the country, educating audiences about these topics. In that time, we wrote the first edition of this book, presented over one thousand programs, and as demand increased, established a team
of incredibly talented sex educators who now copresent our programs.

We teach about many different sexuality-related topics, including consent, communication, LGBTQ issues, and sexual health. Attendees of our "Sex in the Dark"
program submit questions about any sexuality topic under the sun (or the moon,
as the case may be), which we answer on the spot, concluding with a lightning
round of rapid-fire answers. We've fielded thousands and thousands of questions,

but we haven't heard it all. Because sexuality is constantly evolving and changing in response to culture and technology, there's always something new to learn.

But no matter the topic, one theme emerges over and over again: orgasms. There are so many barriers to pleasure, it's left a lot of people wondering why they aren't having orgasms or aren't having them with a partner, or generally feeling that sex should feel better than it actually does. We receive so many mixed-up messages and outright lies about sex, starting with the idea that learning the mechanics of reproduction is somehow more important than learning the ways in which sex can bring joy.

This book fills that gap. We believe you deserve pleasure. Years of feedback from readers of the first edition confirm that pleasure is within reach—sometimes easy reach—as a result of reading these pages. It's the education about orgasms that most people never got in school or from their parents, and certainly didn't get from porn. This is a book about how to have an orgasm if you never have, how to help your partner, how to have multiple orgasms, and everything from squirting to sex toys to anal play to making online sex less awkward. We give you the skinny on topics from faking to penis size to advanced troubleshooting for when your body isn't responding the way you want it to.

People who hear that we educate about sexual pleasure sometimes dismiss it as a breezy, insubstantial topic, or ask questions with a chuckle, like "Can't people figure that out for themselves? I did okay!" Indeed, we *do* try to keep it light-hearted as much as we can. We love a good sex pun as much as anyone; if you can't laugh when you're talking about sex, you're definitely not having enough fun! But look closer, past the joking around, and you quickly see that when it comes to sex, things aren't always so breezy. As much as sex can be something rooted in joy and human connection, it can also be tied to life's worst elements: shame, fear, confusion, and outright lies. Sex can reflect the ugliness of racism, sexism, homophobia, transphobia, and stereotypes galore. There's violence, abuse, and the reality of sexual assault, and the wounds that too many people carry from times when their right to decide about access to their own body was violated. There's the warped fun house mirror of porn, which reflects and distorts our cultural images of sex in powerful and sometimes unexpected ways, even as it entertains and arouses.

We've devoted our professional careers to trying to help people navigate this complicated terrain. And we've seen how helping people become knowledgeable about and comfortable with their own body can transform their daily experience—and, as Dorian discovered firsthand, can even save their life.

Dorian's Story

WHEN I WAS twenty-six years old, I was diagnosed with breast cancer. I didn't have a family history or a single risk factor for the disease (in fact, a doctor later told me my statistical risk of getting breast cancer was *below* average). My cancer wasn't diagnosed by mammogram; people in their twenties don't get routine mammograms. It wasn't discovered through breast self-exam; like many women, I knew I should do them but generally forgot. It wasn't discovered by my gynecologist, who had examined my breasts just a month earlier and declared all was well. Instead, I noticed the lump myself, lying in bed one night and stretching, then absentmindedly running a hand down my arm and across my chest. I wasn't too worried because I knew that most young people's breast lumps turn out to be nothing. I ate healthy foods, I didn't smoke, I had a great relationship with Marshall; things were going so well in my life that my little lump didn't concern me in the least.

As luck would have it, I had an appointment with my doctor a month later, and I mentioned the lump to her. After examining it, she said, "You know, Dorian, I think it's probably nothing, but I'm not one hundred percent sure; let's have some tests done." Still utterly unconcerned, I met with a breast surgeon for an ultrasound and biopsy.

A few days later, the surgeon left a message asking me to call her back. I did, giving the receptionist my name, and she put me on hold for the doctor. Minutes passed as I watched the January snow fall outside my window. The receptionist came back on and said, "I'm so sorry to keep you waiting, Dorian. I know the doctor really wants to talk to you."

At this point, my memory switched to slow motion, like the moments before a car accident when you can see the impact coming but can't do anything to prevent it. I knew the doctor wouldn't feel so urgently about talking to me if the news were good. When she told me my lump was breast cancer, I was flabbergasted. I called Marshall, and he left work early. I picked him up at the commuter train station near our apartment. While snow fell around the car, we put our arms around each other in our puffy winter parkas, so thick we couldn't feel the bodies beneath, and we sobbed.

It's an understatement to say that being diagnosed with cancer is terrifying. It changes your life forever. When I look back, one conclusion resurfaces over and over: Thank God, I hadn't internalized the messages that it's bad or dirty to touch your own body. I particularly thank my parents for raising me to be comfortable in my body. I found my cancer early because I touched my own body without even thinking about it, and because I'd done the same thing enough times before that I noticed a very small change in my breast. If I hadn't, who knows how many weeks, months, or even years might have gone by until someone noticed I had cancer in my breast—and whether I'd still be alive today.

On average, young people's breast cancers are diagnosed far later than older people's, and, as a result, the death rate is far higher—in part because the cancers typically go unnoticed for so long. Helping us make peace with our body and our sexuality isn't just an incidental nicety—in some cases, it can be lifesaving. Two decades later, and counting myself lucky enough to have given birth to (and breastfed!) two healthy children, I'm in remission and doing great. With breast cancer, no doctor will ever tell you that you're "cured." But even though I can't know what the future holds, I feel very, very lucky.

Surviving cancer fuels my passion for educating about sexuality. But it was an earlier experience—learning how to have an orgasm—that first sparked my interest. That didn't happen until shortly after my twentieth birthday.

I was a kid who didn't masturbate while growing up. I knew what masturbation was, and my parents were the liberal types who clearly communicated that touching yourself was okay as long as you were in private (not in the sandbox!). But my limited explorations didn't impress me enough to continue, so I led a happy little-kid existence without masturbation. Didn't do it, didn't think about it, didn't wonder whether other kids were doing it.

The years went by. My mom is a regular reader of the advice column "Dear Abby," and when I was a teenager, she ordered me a copy of Abby's booklet *What Every Teen Should Know*. The booklet, still available to readers today, was full of advice on subjects like dating, drinking, smoking, and other topics of interest to teens, and when I read through the copy my mom gave me, it all seemed quite sensible.

One section worried me, though: the part about masturbation. On this subject, Abby said, "This will be the shortest chapter in the booklet. Why? It is normal. Every healthy, normal person masturbates."

My adult self applauds Abby for sending such an unambiguously positive message about masturbation. But sitting on my bed in my pink-flowered bedroom, the teenage me read and reread that sentence, "Every healthy, normal person masturbates." I knew that Abby's advice track record was stellar. If she said that every healthy, *normal* person masturbates, and I never did, I could come to only one conclusion: there must be something very, very wrong with me.

Even with this new concern, I didn't try masturbating; my sexual urges and impulses didn't truly blossom for a few more years. Since my late-blooming self wasn't touching herself, and my high school romantic life was close to nonexistent, I certainly wasn't having orgasms.

A few years later, I went away to college. At Brown University, where Marshall and I met, there was a dean who gave an annual presentation on masturbation; it was something of a tradition. My sophomore year, I saw a poster on a bulletin board about the upcoming program and said to myself, "I think I need to go to that." The dean's talk fascinated me, and at the end, I left with the resource sheet she had distributed.

Afterward, I walked right to the campus bookstore and plunked down $5.99 to buy the only one of the books on the dean's resource list that was on the shelf that day. Over the next few months, I began to do the exercises in the book, and later that semester, I had my first orgasm. It was the best $5.99 I've ever spent!

As you might imagine, I was thrilled. Ecstatic! And amazed that I was twenty years old before I discovered that my body could do this incredible thing. I couldn't believe it had been so easy to learn. Intrigued, I set out to learn everything I could about orgasms, whiling away hours in the university library reading every journal article on the subject that I could locate. I started writing about what I was learning—first papers for classes, then articles for a wider audience. I pursued training as a sex educator while I was a student, and when I started dating Marshall, who was also studying sexuality as an academic subject, it seemed only natural that we'd continue the learning process together. Soon, we began teaching sexuality workshops.

There's no question we have seen massive advances in gender equality in the last half century. But for those who, like me, were assigned female at birth and grew up surrounded by cultural messages about what it means to be a girl, sexuality is still stuck in a surprising paradox. We experience a culture happy to sell revealing, "sexy" clothes (to ever-younger ages), but that still doesn't explain where to find the clitoris. While kids with a penis usually figure out how to bring themselves to orgasm by age thirteen, half of us with a clitoris don't have our first orgasm until our late teens, twenties, or beyond. Among teens and college students, oral sex on penises is to be expected, while those with a vagina have often heard so much vile cunnilingus slang that they're too insecure to receive the same kind of pleasure. It's still a radical act to say that young people need and deserve access to information about their *own sexual pleasure*—not just about the risks and negative consequences of sex.

Marshall's Story

SURE, WE LEARNED about sexuality in my middle school and high school sex education classes. What did we learn about? Fallopian tubes! Generations of us have the classic diagram burned into our brain as if *that's* the most important thing we all need to know about sex. Breaking: If you didn't know fallopian tubes existed, you'd probably be just fine—nothing bad would happen. No one will ever whisper seductively into your ear, "Ooh, babe, will you stroke my fallopian tubes?"

Yet the clitoris, an organ far more important to most people's future lives, was always mysteriously missing from those sex ed diagrams. I can only imagine how life might be different if the image burned into our brain was not the fallopian tubes but the location of the clitoris. Now *that* would be useful for so many of us! The problems with the way sex ed is taught in most high schools really hit home for me when I saw my friends taking driver's ed. Driver's ed is an eminently practical class, complete with those cars with DANGER: STUDENT DRIVER signs on the roof. In driver's ed, they teach you how to drive.

Sometimes I'd think about what it would be like if driver's ed were taught the way sex ed is. You would show up in the classroom (there would definitely *not* be a student driver car), and the teacher would say, "Welcome to driver's ed. You need to know that driving is very, *very* dangerous. You could die! So don't drive. Just don't do it—until you're married. If you absolutely *insist* on driving, wear a seat belt." After this, you'd spend a bit of time practicing putting a seat belt on a banana, and then class would be dismissed and your driver's education would be considered complete. But you'd never actually learn how to drive a car: where to find the gas pedal, how to turn on the headlights, or even how to back it out of a driveway.

Looking to fill those knowledge gaps, both for myself and others, has turned into a career. I started as a writer for my college newspaper, volunteering to cover any event on campus relating to sexuality: workshops on body image, rallies against sexual assault, and panels on LGBTQ issues. Halfway through college, the university announced a new interdisciplinary major, Sexuality and Society, and I signed right up. Soon, I was hired to write an online sex column for a Barnes & Noble website. The more I studied and wrote about sex, the more people shared with me stories of their own experiences and asked me questions. I was blown away by the incredible range of people's sexual thoughts, feelings, and experiences.

When Dorian and I started dating, learning became a joint project since she, too, had training as a sex educator. We'd attend sexuality conferences together and buy each other books to discuss. Little by little, we started writing articles together, facilitating support groups, and giving workshops at conferences and adult education centers about relationships, sex, and LGBTQ issues. For six years after college, I managed HIV prevention programs at a busy community health center in Boston, where I founded a safer sex educator team, training volunteers to talk to people in the city's bars and clubs about reducing their sexual risks.

Before long, Dorian and I started fielding requests from college students who'd heard us at conferences and wanted to bring us to speak at their university. Since then it's taken on a life of its own. Whether it's at a college in the heartland surrounded by cornfields; a lecture hall in Ankara, Turkey; or a corporate webinar on sexual wellness for a global company, our audiences are hungry to learn.

It's truly been an honor to hear from readers and audience members that something we wrote or taught was life changing. Maybe it was figuring out how to have an orgasm for the first time, or getting up the courage to tell a partner about a fantasy and make it a reality. I'll never forget a note from a woman who'd attended one of our presentations years earlier. That night, she and her boyfriend had the best and most honest conversation about their sex life that they'd ever had, including what she needed to feel safe and experience pleasure as a sexual assault survivor. She said that conversation had been transformative for their relationship, and they had progressed from dating to being happily married. I continue to be honored and humbled every day doing this work.

Introducing Maybe Burke

THIS BOOK WAS originally published with the title *I ♥ Female Orgasm: An Extraordinary Orgasm Guide*. This new edition's title reflects the book's inclusion of trans and nonbinary people.

The first edition of the book was groundbreaking at the time. No book devoted to "female" orgasm included as many trans experiences and perspectives. It included a section specifically about orgasms for transgender folks, a section for partners of trans people, and quotes throughout from the transgender people who had participated in the book's survey. The book was widely praised for its inclusiveness.

But sex education is not a static field; it's constantly evolving. This keeps us sex educators on our toes and also makes an updated edition of this book feel imperative. In this new edition, we're thrilled to have Maybe Burke, a fellow sex educator and a transgender advocate, as a coauthor of this book. The three of us have fundamentally revised how every paragraph of the book addresses gender, anatomy, and orgasms. Orgasms and sexual pleasure for transgender and nonbinary people have moved out of their own chapter and been woven into every chapter, sometimes in the main text, sometimes in sections that highlight angles that may be of particular interest to trans and nonbinary readers. You'll find Maybe's wisdom for trans people and their partners throughout these pages.

Maybe's Story

[Content note: The first half of this section includes mentions of sexual violence.]

I didn't really understand that I was trans until I was nineteen years old, when I first started learning about words and experiences that would later be considered to fall under the nonbinary umbrella. (At the time, *nonbinary* wasn't yet a word I was hearing people use.) Today, I consider myself in both the transgender and nonbinary categories. I cannot speak on behalf of all trans and nonbinary people (nor would I want to), and I acknowledge that there are transgender people who aren't nonbinary and nonbinary people who don't consider themselves transgender. We'll be using the phrase *trans and nonbinary* quite often in the pages that follow, though, to acknowledge the breadth of experiences and identities we're talking about. I don't think anything we'll say will literally be true for all trans and nonbinary people; rather, something to consider if you or your partner are not cisgender.

While I was a teenager, still unaware of my gender identity and fumbling to understand my sexuality and sexual orientation, I was an ongoing victim of sexual assault. I know there are many people who don't like to use the word *victim* for a number of reasons, but it's the word I use to describe myself at fourteen years old, being abused by a man in his twenties. I grew up performing in community theaters, and he worked at one of them. He preyed on young performers who wanted attention and had bad relationships with their parents. For me, this abuse lasted until I went away to college and it had a significant impact on the ways I viewed sex and pleasure in the years that followed. I had no concept of what consent was supposed to look like, no basis for how sex was supposed to connect to emotional intimacy, and no understanding of my own

> ## Definitions, Please?
>
> **Nonbinary:** Anyone who does not identify exclusively within the binary of being a man or a woman.
>
> **Transgender (sometimes shortened to "trans"):** Anyone whose sex assigned at birth doesn't match their gender identity.
>
> **Cisgender (sometimes shortened to "cis"):** Anyone whose gender identity matches their sex assigned at birth.
>
> **Sex assigned at birth:** Shortly after you were born, an adult in the room (probably doctor, midwife, or one of your parents) glanced at your genitals and said, "It's a boy!" or "It's a girl!"

desires or wants. Sex, as I understood it, was just a thing that would happen to me, not a thing I could initiate or even invite. I now recognize what I was experiencing was rape, not sex, but it colored my understanding and interrupted all my early experiences.

As I grew up and changed the ways I looked at both my gender and sexuality, I realized that so many of my life experiences were not commonly discussed. Some of the things that were most important to me were things you never really heard conversations about or saw reflected in movie plots. (This was before Laverne Cox was on the cover of *Time* magazine, associated with the "Transgender Tipping Point" and before the #MeToo movement.) So, I decided to start telling my stories and sharing my experiences. I talked about the things that were taboo to mention. I found that the more I talked, the more people agreed and shared their similar experiences. Talking about my experiences and claiming myself as a survivor of sexual assault helped others realize that similar things that had happened to them were also not okay. Claiming my gender identity and choosing a name for myself helped other trans and nonbinary people feel seen and valid within their identities. I learned very quickly that talking about the things we're taught to ignore or suppress is actually incredibly freeing, and can be a part of changing someone's world.

I started having those conversations louder and more publicly, shaping a career as an advocate. A lot of the work that I did, and still do today, is listening. Most of what I know is simply from embedding myself within communities, hearing the language people are using, and amplifying what they want those outside the community to know. I read books by trans and nonbinary elders, I learn our histories, and I stay tuned into what communities are asking and fighting for today. This work and this learning is ongoing and constant, but I found that marrying my love of storytelling with my passion for social justice made me an effective advocate. I founded the Trans Literacy Project—a collaboration with trans artists, advocates, and activists to create an accessible web series about trans experiences from the perspective of trans people—and became a trainer for the Philadelphia-based Transgender Training Institute, offering professional development and personal growth trainings on trans and nonbinary inclusion. In all my work, I focus on expanding conversations for people who are often left out and marginalized, specifically around gender.

I started working with Marshall and Dorian, both helping to make sure all of their programming was as inclusive and expansive as possible in terms of gender, and copresenting programs on LGBTQ topics at colleges and universities around the country. I try to center joy in most of my work, so it brings *me* joy to be able to bring this advocacy and inclusion to a book that centers pleasure in such a direct and intentional way.

A Note About Language

THIS SECOND EDITION represents our best effort to write accurately and inclusively about an extraordinary diversity of experiences. One thing that's become apparent to us in decades of doing our best to teach inclusively is that linguistic rules and expectations, especially relating to trans and nonbinary experiences, evolve with sometimes dizzying speed. Since the first edition was published in 2007, words like *cisgender* and *nonbinary* that were hardly used or known have become commonplace. (Julia Serrano's book *Whipping Girl*, which popularized the term *cisgender*, was published in May 2007, three months after *I ♥ Female Orgasm*.)

As a result of these kinds of linguistic changes since the first edition, we've updated the language we use to better reflect the current understanding that not everyone who has a vagina is a woman, and not every woman has a vagina. And likewise, not everyone who has a penis is a man, and not every man has a penis. When we're writing about gender identity, we use words like *man, woman, transgender,* and *nonbinary.* When we're writing about anatomy, we use such phrases as *people with a vagina, people with a penis, vagina-owners,* and *penis-owners.*

In case there's any question, the only person who "owns" a vagina is the person whose body that vagina is part of! Ditto for a penis. A partner can adore and celebrate your genitals, but they sure as heck don't own them.

You'll also see the phrases *people with a vulva* and *people with a vagina.* In general, *vulva* is the more inclusive term, encompassing an entire set of genitalia, not just one part, so mostly the book will refer to vulvas. However, when discussing vagina-specific activities, like vaginal penetration or G-spot stimulation, we'll shift the language accordingly.

Exceptions to This Book's Inclusive Language

THERE ARE TWO types of places in this edition where you'll notice a departure from our general rules. The first are the quotes throughout the book. We love how quotes from our surveys bring many voices and myriad perspectives and experiences into the book, not just our own. To be true to these voices, we include quotes as they were written, including the pronouns (most are writing about real partners whose pronouns are known). If a person writes about the "women" or "men" they've dated, their words are included unchanged; we trust that these words accurately reflect the identities of the people being described.

While those who filled out our survey were of all sexual orientations, on some topics, the cisgender heterosexual respondents reported more difficulties, and therefore had far more to say, than did the LGBTQ respondents. You'll see a lot of gendered language in those quotes as people wrote from their personal experience.

The second situation where you'll see more gendered language is in our descriptions of research studies and historical data. Most studies report their findings in terms of "women" and "men," and few explain their procedure if a transgender person applies to take part in the study. (Would the data from a trans masculine research participant with a vagina have been counted as a man to match his identity? As a woman because of anatomy? Or would this person have been excluded from participating in the study, or dropped from the data?) After spending some time wrestling with how to report binary research findings inclusively, we concluded our best option would be to carry forward the language used in that study. It would not surprise us if the way research is carried out and reported evolves before this book's third edition!

We're well aware that using these phrases is not a perfect solution, even if they are the best we've got for now, in part because of the complexity of bodies and identities. We'll address the ways in which both anatomy and identity, separately and together, can impact people's experience of pleasure and orgasm, and try to do so using the most inclusive language possible.

Another linguistic change since 2007 is the use of gender-expansive pronouns. While the first edition referred to people with a vulva as *she*, people with a penis as *he*, and partners of any gender as *he or she*, this new edition uses *they* for all these situations unless we are writing about a specific person whose pronoun is *he* or *she*.

We are humble about our attempt to shift this entire book toward inclusive language—we know there will be places where some people feel that we didn't get it exactly right and could have been more inclusive. There will be those who feel we went overboard in our efforts. Unquestionably, as the years go by, some of the language in this book, which accurately reflected best practices to the best of our ability at the moment the manuscript left our hands, will become outdated. If at the time you're reading this book, your body or your life doesn't fit neatly into the language we use, we encourage you to make the substitutions needed so our words make sense for you. The basic principles taught here transcend the specific language choices.

Racial Injustice as a Barrier

OUR COUNTRY'S UNDERSTANDING of the impact of racism on sexuality has also evolved since the first edition of this book. As white authors of this book, it's important to acknowledge that this country has an appalling, unforgivable history of trying to control Black and brown people's bodies, reproduction, and sexuality. Those traumas and scars are still present today. Our country has failed to provide the education and the options so that young people of color can be empowered to make the best choices for their own future—including the right to access sexual pleasure on their own terms.

Racism has limited Black and brown students' access to sex education. Black students nationwide are far more likely than white students to receive abstinence-only sex education, according to research published in the *Washington University*

Law Review. Abstinence-only is an approach to sex education that's shame based and one-size-fits-all. It teaches that the only acceptable path is no sex until you're married and involves withholding other information from students. Now, there's no question that abstinence can be a great option for students and for adults in many life stages. But it's never going to be the path that's right for all unmarried adults. As a result of this approach, in the US Black students on average receive less sexuality information than white students.

So often, the US looks at issues like teen pregnancy, HIV, or sexually transmitted infections (STIs), and points to youth of color as being "high-risk groups," as if communities of color are the problem, instead of addressing the ways that *racism* is the problem. The legacy of systemic racism means that youth of color are far more likely to live in poverty, have limited access to health care and sexual health services, and understandably distrust the medical system than their white counterparts.

Many activists, scholars, and sex educators of color are bringing awareness and change around this issue. We're particularly inspired by those making the connections to pleasure, like adrienne maree brown, who wrote, "Pleasure—embodied, connected pleasure—is one of the ways we know when we are free. That we are always free. That we always have the power to co-create the world. Pleasure helps us move through times that are unfair, through grief and loneliness, through the terror of genocide, or days when the demands are just overwhelming. Pleasure heals the places where our hearts and spirit get wounded. Pleasure reminds us that even in the dark, we are alive. Pleasure is a medicine for the suffering that is absolutely promised in life."

Our Survey: The Best Insights Are from Readers Like You

AT THE HEART of this book is a detailed survey that 1,569 people (evidence that the universe has a sense of humor?) took the time to fill out, and share their experiences and advice. This is in addition to the 1,956 who filled out a similar survey for the first edition. The survey data is reflected throughout the book in people's own words (italicized quotes), in statistics and charts, and in our advice. Thanks to this valuable information source, what you'll find in the pages ahead isn't just our opinion or advice from some scientist in a research laboratory. It's reality-tested against the experiences of 3,525 people, at least some of whom are likely a lot like you.

Given that transgender and nonbinary people are underrepresented and even ignored in other research studies, Maybe developed additional survey questions specifically for transgender and nonbinary people, and we made a special effort to recruit transgender and nonbinary participants. In the new survey, 343 trans and nonbinary people responded to the survey, as did 1,226 cisgender people. Eighty-seven percent of survey respondents were from the United States and represented all fifty states. The remaining 13 percent came from thirty-seven countries around the world.

The data and quotes throughout the book reflect incredible diversity of every kind. In some quotes, it may be apparent that the person is disabled, intersex, Black, trans masculine, demiromantic, a sexual assault survivor, Christian, kinky, or *many* other identities. However, in other cases, there is no way to guess at the person's identity based on the observation or experience they shared.

This book draws on data and wisdom from other sources. With our colleague Lindsay Fram, we conducted in-depth focus groups with students at colleges, private and public, small and large, all around the country, from California to Virginia. We learned so much from these participants as they sorted through for us what sex and hookups mean for them and their generation.

We also learned a lot from the 282 Pure Romance consultants who filled out our survey on sex toys. You'll see more on them in Chapter 7. And this book is all the wiser thanks to a team of research assistants pulling journal articles, colleagues consulting on specific issues, and expert readers, whose names appear in the acknowledgments but whose gift of knowledge is on every page.

What Else Is New in This Edition?

ALTHOUGH BODY PARTS work the same way now as they did when the first edition came out fifteen years ago, the world around us has changed a great deal.

We've gone through every chapter with a fine-tooth comb, updated data to reflect the latest research, and made lots of additions throughout, including:

- Some major advances in sex toys
- An updated explanation of squirting based on the newest research findings
- Advice on making online and digital sex less awkward
- A history-of-the-vibrator story from the first edition that turns out to have been a tall tale
- Expanded exploration of the role porn plays in people's lives, especially as they come of age
- Lots more content about penises, prostates, and related activities as part of the expanded vision of who this book is for
- More information for and about asexual people
- Expanded content about consent throughout the book, including tips on making consent navigation less awkward and more comfortable
- More discussion of body image as it relates to sexual pleasure
- Great new tools, such as body tours
- An updated and expanded list of woman- and LGBTQ-owned/friendly sex toy stores around the world
- Information about some medical diagnoses that can work against sexual pleasure, including vaginismus and vulvodynia
- The addition of a book website where you'll find links to a host of websites, books, and social media accounts to explore topics in more depth. Moving these online, out of the book's pages, will allow us to keep the list more up-to-date and add new recommendations that readers share (we hope you'll tell us your favorites!).

Beyond the Big O

ALTHOUGH IT MAY sound more than a little ironic, given the topic of this book, if you think sex is just about orgasms, you're missing out.

Here's the thing: orgasms are really, *really* fun. They feel great; in fact, they're likely to be one of the most pleasurable physical sensations you'll ever experience. For many people, they rank way up there as emotional and spiritual experiences too.

But orgasms aren't the only point of sex. Get too obsessed with orgasms, and you can miss out on a lot of other things: The sensations of touching and being touched. The experience of riding the roller coaster of arousal with its teasing climb and unexpected surges. The quieter joy of intimacy. As the best partners know, you can have great sex without an orgasm at all.

We've seen orgasm obsession lead people astray. Often this happens when a couple has a single sexual experience in which an expected orgasm didn't happen: a lost erection for no reason whatsoever; or not being able to come through oral sex, even though that had always worked before. Some turn to us in these moments with a feeling of panic: Does my partner still find me sexy? Does he still love me? What's wrong with me, with her, with him, with them, with us? The greater the panic, the more tension the next time they have sex. The more tense they are, the less chance of future orgasms. The downward spiral begins.

That's why each individual orgasm isn't the point. If you have an orgasm on a given night, great! If not, laugh. Or sigh. It's not a big deal, and the journey can be as sweet as the destination. There's too much fun, pleasure, and intimacy to be had—by yourself or with someone else—to spend a lot of energy worrying about any individual orgasm.

We were moved by the words of the person who typed at the end of their survey:

I hope you'll include a message that it's OK not to want orgasms, or to decide they're not worth the effort, instead of contributing to the chorus trying to make me feel broken.

We'll say it loud and clear: You are not broken. It's absolutely okay not to want orgasms or to decide they're not worth the effort. You—each and every person reading this book—get to decide what role, if any, orgasms will have in your life. Your answer is likely to change, possibly many times, as the years pass. Read this book not only for advice about how to reach the orgasmic finish line but also about how to enjoy good sex if that's something you want. Listen to your own body, relax, have fun, and be true to your own needs and desires (as long as they don't harm you or anyone else).

Last but not least, if anything we say contradicts the experience of the naked person in your bed, believe them. Each person knows their own body better than we possibly could.

1

The Lowdown on the Big O

TOP TEN REASONS TO HAVE AN ORGASM

1. It feels great.
2. It's free.
3. It's legal.
4. It reduces stress.
5. It's good for your heart, skin, and brain.
6. It helps you fall asleep.
7. It can help relieve menstrual cramps and headaches.
8. It might help you live longer.
9. It's available to you whether you have a partner or not.
10. Why not?!?

BONUS: There's nothing else quite like it.

What Is an Orgasm, Anyway?

ONCE YOU STRIP away the romance and open-mouthed shrieks of pleasure (or the silent, blissful tremor of a quieter orgasm), an orgasm is just a sudden release of sexual tension. You can't control how an orgasm feels, just as you can't exactly control the sensation of a sneeze. (Let us guess: Did you, too, have that kids' book about sexuality that describes an orgasm as being like a sneeze? If so, we bet you were pleasantly surprised when your first orgasm felt nothing like a sneeze!) During arousal, the bloodstream is spiked with pleasurable hormones, like oxytocin, and at the moment of orgasm, even more flood in. It's your body's best natural high.

During an orgasm, many people (but not all) feel muscles contract in their vagina and uterus, the base of their penis, and/or their anus, and sometimes in other parts of their body, like their hands and feet. Some people describe a sensation like waves of warmth washing over their genitals or over their whole body; some say it feels like lightning bolts of electricity. An orgasm can happen in quiet stillness or with lots of bodily movements.

I feel warm. My body stiffens and, with a particularly strong orgasm, my face tingles and my legs stop working.

My breath catches, I either can't make a sound, or I'm stifling a scream (thin walls in my apartment complex). My entire body goes rigid, my toes curl, my fingers clutch at whatever happens to be handy, and I shudder. I generally can't move.

It's like this unbelievable, almost unbearable buildup of tension and almost too much pleasure till I just feel like my whole body is struggling and squirming for some sort of release. And then suddenly it's like something just breaks free and I feel tingles all over and sort of an electric buzz. Then I just feel calm and relaxed.

Although being highly sexually aroused is extremely pleasurable in its own right, an orgasm is (usually) a short period where the intensity of pleasurable sensation is much higher than in the arousal period just before. Most orgasms last three to twenty-two seconds although it's possible for them to last a minute or more for some people with a vulva. There are big, strong, wowwowwowWOW! orgasms, barely noticeable ones, and everything in between. Orgasms vary from person to person and from orgasm to orgasm. Each orgasm is unique—like a snowflake!

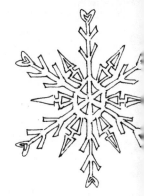

It feels so good I forget about everything else in the world for a few seconds. It just feels like being alive, with every cell vibrating.

I used to call my orgasms mini-O's because I thought orgasms were going to be better, more body-shaking, if you know what I mean. But then I came to accept the fact that this is it. But I'm learning to enjoy it more, so it's okay.

An orgasm can feel almost spiritual, complete, like I'm one with my partner.

The Almighty Clitoris

YOU PROBABLY ALREADY know that for most people who have one, the clitoris (pronounced KLIT-eh-rus or kli-TOR-es—either way is correct) is the primary sex organ. Whereas a penis is a multiuse tool—it can be used for reproduction, urination, and pleasure, pleasure is the clitoris's only reason for existence. Research finds that although the penis and clitoris grow from the same tissue in the early development of a fetus, the clitoris is the

more sensitive organ. The head of the clit has more nerve endings per square inch than any other part of human anatomy, and two to four times more than the head of a penis.

> ### "Coming" Versus "Having an Orgasm"
>
> WHEN SOMEONE CRIES out, "I'm coming!" does that mean they are about to have an orgasm or about to ejaculate? If they have a penis, those two things usually go hand in hand, so if your partner with a penis says, "I'm about to come!" consider it a heads-up that ejaculate, or "cum," is on the way.
>
> If you have a clitoris, "I'm coming!" simply means "I'm having an orgasm!" There doesn't need to be any ejaculating, or "squirting," involved. (If you're like, "Hold on, ejaculation for someone with a clitoris?" check out Chapter 6, where we'll explain everything.)

Hold the Morphine, Give Me an Orgasm

RESEARCHERS WHO STUDY clitoris owners in laboratories find that their sensitivity to pain is dramatically reduced when they're aroused, and even lower during an orgasm. Several studies have first determined how much pressure a person found painful under normal circumstances (for instance, by pressing on their finger). When the same person was sexually aroused, these studies found they could comfortably experience significantly more pressure before they said it was too painful. During orgasm, the pressure could be far more intense (more than twice as much in some cases) before they found it too much to tolerate.

It's not just that orgasms distract us from pain, either, because other distracting activities don't have the same pain-relieving results. MRIs show that orgasms release endorphins and naturally occurring steroids that temporarily numb the nerve endings that signal pain.

Many people with a clitoris find that this lovely feature outlasts the climax itself. Some say having an orgasm reduces the intensity of their menstrual cramps, and others have found significant headache relief from having an orgasm. One woman told us she'd discovered that orgasm was the surest way to end a migraine. She laughed that, while other women might use the phrase, "Honey, I have a headache," as a way to dodge their partners' advances, her partner knows that if she uses the identical sentence, she's initiating a night of passion.

Starting in the 1970s, researchers and groups of self-taught clitoris-owners began to take a closer look at this body part. They pointed out that rather than just being a tiny nub, the entire organ has eighteen separate parts, many of them internal and some quite large. In addition to the glans, shaft, hood, and inner lips (the clit's primary externally visible parts, which you can see on page 61), inside the body there is also a pair of wishbone-shaped clitoral legs made of erectile tissue. These are 2 to 3½ inches long, point back toward the tailbone, and fill with blood during arousal.

Bulbs of erectile tissue lie under the inner lips, and erectile tissue also surrounds the urethra, the tube you pee through. (This area, the urethral sponge, is also called the G-spot. For more on this, and a diagram of how this all fits together inside the body, see Chapter 6.) The clitoral organ also includes a complex of nerves, blood vessels, muscles, ligaments, and glands that assist in lubrication and, in some cases, ejaculation.

What does this all mean? First, it means a clitoris's potential for sexual pleasure is quite expansive—far more than the little "button" many of us learned about. Yet the clit doesn't always get the attention it deserves. Health textbooks sometimes neglect to include or label the clitoris in their anatomy diagrams. (Can you imagine a diagram of genital anatomy omitting the penis?)

The word *vagina* regularly steals some of the clit's limelight. When parents try to teach their children the correct anatomical terms, they often use the words *penis* and *vagina*. While those terms are accurate, they are not equivalent! Many children with a clitoris grow up with no idea that they have this body part (and rarely learn the word *vulva*, the actual word for the collection of external organs many see when they look between their legs). The widespread use of the word *vagina* is a major step forward, given that not long ago, the part called "hoo-hoo," "coochie," or just "down there" couldn't be named in polite company. Perhaps someday, the lusty, trusty clitoris will get its own day to shine. Looking to meet your clit? Check out pages 60–63.

Leave it to the artists!

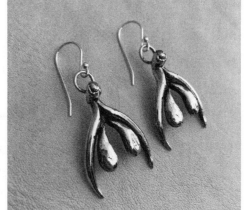

Thanks to Spring Winders, who creates clitoris-themed jewelry, you can now dangle your favorite body part from your earlobes.

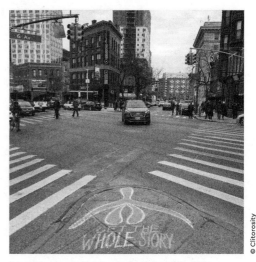

Laura Kingsley and her team of artists at Clitorosity educate in the most unexpected places about the true shape of the clitoris.

Arousal: How Does It Work?

MASTERS AND JOHNSON, the pioneering sex researcher couple of the 1950s and '60s, studied sexual arousal in their laboratory back when hooking people up to machines and watching them masturbate or have sex was pretty radical. (Okay, so it still is!) Based on what they learned from their observations, they described what they called the "human sexual response cycle." Some contemporary experts criticize various aspects of Masters and Johnson's work, including the way it's overly simplistic, as if sex always flowed directly from arousal to orgasm without variation. Despite their shortcomings, lots of people today find Masters and Johnson's concepts helpful in understanding their own sexual response.

What's Between *Your* Legs?

OUR SURVEY ASKED people what words their parents used for sexual parts while they were growing up. Although most parents used terms like *vagina* or *penis*, and many others didn't ever discuss those parts of the body, some parents got pretty creative. Here are some of the words respondents told us their parents used:

Instead of vagina or vulva:

between-the-legs birdie	down there
book ("Keep your book closed so no one else can read it.")	flower
	fluffy
choo-choo	giny (rhymes with "shiny")
coochie coo	hoo-hoo
cookie jar	hoosie
coolie	king-king
coos	muffin

mutzie

papaya

pat-a-cake

pee-tu

pizza

pom-pom

private area

putterpat

snuffleupagus

special area

tinkler

tu-tu

tulip

twittle

wee

The penis earns its own set of euphemisms:

birdie

bits

coocoo

dangly bits

ding-a-ling

ding-dong

dingle

joe

johnson

monster

Mr. Turtle

no-no area

nuggets

pecker

pee-pee

peenga

peeper

peeshcadell (with Italian dad
    accent)

pickle

pishy

pito

tallywacker

thingaling

ting

tottie

wee-wee

weiner

willywinky

winkie dinkie

wooper

The classic Masters and Johnson cycle begins with the excitement phase (though newer theories of arousal point out that sexual desire often, but not always, comes before excitement). In the excitement phase, the fun begins: Typically, your heart starts beating faster, breathing and blood pressure increase; blood flows to the genitals; your vagina might start to get wet, or lubricate. Both clitorises *and* penises get bigger and harder as people get turned on. Some people experience a "sex flush" of pink or darker skin on their neck, chest, or other parts of their body. Your nipples might become erect, and if you have vaginal lips, both the inner and outer ones may swell. Most of the time, you aren't thinking about or even aware of the changes in your body. You're just thinking, "Yeah, this feels *good*!"

Then, said Masters and Johnson, there's a plateau phase. You're at a higher level of arousal than you normally are, but for some people it feels like they got stuck, as if they're no longer making progress. Although some later theorists of sexual response omit this phase from their models of arousal, many vulva-owners, in particular, tell us it describes their experience perfectly. Before Dorian had ever had an orgasm, she'd get aroused, and then get frustrated when it seemed like nothing was happening. So, she'd just give up trying, disappointed, and conclude, "I must be broken." Reading about the plateau phase was her number one break-through to having an orgasm; she was stunned to learn that *most* people with a vulva experience a plateau phase. If that's the case, she concluded, it meant her going-nowhere arousal wasn't a sign she was broken—it was a sign she was *normal*. Some days, a person may slip directly from excitement to orgasm with barely a plateau phase at all, while other days, you might feel that you're stuck in plateau land forever.

Most of the time, if the stimulation continues that got you to the plateau phase in the first place,

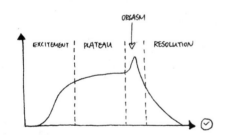

Masters and Johnson drew the plateau phase like this…

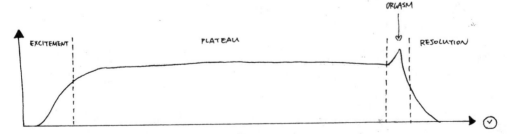

…but if it takes you a long time to have an orgasm, sometimes it can feel more like this.

Tick, Tick, Tick, BOOM!

ON AVERAGE, IT takes a person with a clitoris twenty minutes of direct clitoral stimulation to have an orgasm when they're with a partner. The average penis-owner: two to five minutes. It's definitely not fair! We'd start an online petition to have this changed if only we could figure out where to send it once it has a billion signatures.

Keep in mind that twenty minutes is an *average*. Potentially half of clitoris-owners take longer than twenty minutes to have an orgasm. Thirty minutes, forty minutes (or more!) is not unusual.

Of course, the reverse can also be true. Some people with a clitoris come very quickly, and some people with a penis take a long time.

Perhaps most interesting of all: When a person is enjoying some self-love without a partner around, the length of time to orgasm is about the same regardless of genitals. It seems to be the presence of the partner that slows down the average orgasm time for vaginas. In most cases, partners aren't as effective at stimulating a clit as the clit's owner is. Maybe clit-owners get self-conscious or tend to shift their attention to giving rather than receiving pleasure. Maybe being with a partner distracts our brain or our body from that straight path to orgasmic glory—even if we love their intimacy and the way they turn us on. Only one thing is certain: it's complicated!

People require varying amounts of stimulation too. We can't say it any better than *The Guide to Getting It On* by Paul Joannides: "Some people have orgasms when a lover kisses them on the back of the neck; others need a stick or two of dynamite between the legs. The amount of stimulation needed to generate an orgasm has nothing to do with how much a person enjoys sex." As with everything related to sex, "normal" is fantastically diverse.

eventually you'll have an orgasm. YAY! Your breathing and heart rate double. Interestingly, brain waves during an intense orgasm resemble the brain waves of a person in deep meditation. People usually like to have the stimulation continue straight through the length of their orgasm. So, if it's your finger, tongue, or penis that's providing the joyride, keep it going until your partner signals you to stop or moves away!

After the climax, there's a resolution phase, during which your body slowly returns to its nonaroused state. That's unless you're having a multiple orgasm day—a lot easier for vulvas than penises. More about this on page 33.

Socks Help

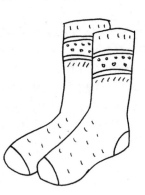

A NOW-FAMOUS STUDY that involved having people masturbate inside an MRI machine found that 80 percent of the men and women wearing socks had orgasms, compared with 50 percent with bare feet. Maybe blood flow is part of the story—a body that doesn't have to direct its blood to try to keep one's feet warm has more blood flowing to the genitals. But that's not the explanation offered by Gert Holstege, the researcher running the study. He said that socks simply helped people feel more comfortable.

Clitoral Troubleshooting: What to Do About a Too-Sensitive Clit?

HERE'S A QUESTION frequently asked by our audience members: "Sometimes my clit (or my partner's clit) gets so sensitive it hurts to be touched. It's as if it skipped over the orgasm and reached the kind of sensitivity I'd expect *after* I have an orgasm. What can I do?" Others describe having their clitoris become numb rather than overly sensitive. If you've had either experience, or your partner has, here are some things you can try:

○ **Try more indirect touching.** For many clit-owners, the head (glans) of the clitoris is too sensitive to touch or may quickly become oversensitive. Try focusing stimulation on only the shaft (that's often the main part they like touched), or other nearby parts of the vulva that might tug or vibrate the skin around the clitoris gently without touching it directly. For some of us, the nerves in the clit are so sensitive that it's best to stimulate it through our fleshy outer lips (fingers on the outside of the outer lips, clit on the inside).

Sometimes I find it's necessary to rub to the side or above or below the clit rather than directly on top of it. It often feels better than the painful sensation that can happen as a result of rubbing directly on the clit.

- **Take lots of mini-breaks.** Some clits respond best to an approach that's a bit like "Two steps forward, take a break, allow arousal to slide back a step, then start up again." Try lots of on-again, off-again clitoral attention, with periods of a few seconds or a few minutes without any clitoral stimulation, until you reach the orgasmic home stretch. (At that point, you'll probably want to stay with it.)
- **Keep it really wet.** If you're touching your (or your partner's) clit with your fingers, keep rewetting with saliva or lube or "dip into the honeypot" frequently (dip your fingers into the vagina, if it's quite wet).
- **Observe the expert.** Partners can study what the clitoris-owner does during masturbation (if they self-pleasure and are comfortable sharing the experience with you). Pay particular attention to how direct or indirect the stimulation is, what kind of motion they're using (up and down, back and forth, circles, most of the focus on one side or the other, etc.), how gentle or hard the pressure is, and how frequently they add wetness.
- **Be gentle.** This is especially true early on. If you're the partner, ask for feedback about whether a lighter touch might help or if your partner would prefer more focus on other body parts.

Grow Your O by Edging

A QUICKIE CAN be perfect sometimes, but in general, the longer the buildup, the bigger the orgasm. If you're getting too close too fast, back off the stimulation and bring yourself back up a few times for bigger fireworks.

I find that when I'm close to orgasm, if I stop and wait a minute or so and then continue, and do this over and over again as a way of teasing myself, when I finally do come, it's a lot more intense.

I ♥ ORGASMS

○ **Recognize that, some days, orgasm is just not meant to be.** Sex (including masturbation) is an imperfect art. Some days, it's glorious; some days, it's "good enough"; some days, it just doesn't work at all. That's not cause for alarm, and definitely not reason to worry that the love is over, or that you and your partner aren't meant for each other. Have a sense of humor, and remember that most people with a vulva can be quite satisfied without an orgasm.

What's Up with Wetness?

AS PEOPLE WITH a vagina get turned on, their vagina usually lubricates, creating sometimes considerable quantities (sometimes not so much) of slippery wetness that can help make touch and penetration feel great. Vaginas can start getting wet within just seconds of the beginning of mental or physical stimulation. Where does this lovely liquid magically appear from? In early arousal, extra blood rushes to the genitals. The lubricating fluid, or transudate, is actually a colorless component of blood. It contains water, pyridine, squalene, urea, acetic acid, lactic acid, complex alcohols and glycols, ketones, and aldehydes. You can't just cook this stuff up with a chemistry set! It's squeezed through the vaginal walls, making the walls of the vagina so nice and slippery.

People often assume the wetness of a vagina is like a neon sign that announces its owner's state of arousal. In fact, how wet you are is a surprisingly *inaccurate* indicator of how turned on you are. The official term for this is *arousal nonconcordance*. Turns out, it's a myth that a wet vagina signifies an aroused vagina-owner. A person can be *super* turned on without much genital response. Conversely, a person's vagina can be dripping wet—but the vagina's owner may not be in the mood for sex. (It actually works the same way for penises. Most penis-owners will attest there are times when they are totally in the mood for sex but have a hard time getting an erection. And most remember some awkward moment trying to hide a poorly timed erection in a nonsexy, nonaroused moment.) This lack of alignment between our brain and our genitals happens to everyone and is entirely normal, but research finds it's way more common for vaginas.

Whether or not the vagina in your life is producing lots of wetness, store-bought lube is one of the world's best inventions. It's more valuable than ever after menopause, when sexual desire may be strong but the body's lubrication typically decreases. See page 166 for more on lube.

There's More to Sex than What's Between Your Legs

SOMETIMES PARTNERS NEED a reminder that there are other erogenous zones besides what's between each other's legs. Here's what our survey (for more on our research, see page 14) found when we asked people their favorite erogenous zones—the places they like to be kissed, licked, and caressed besides their genitals:

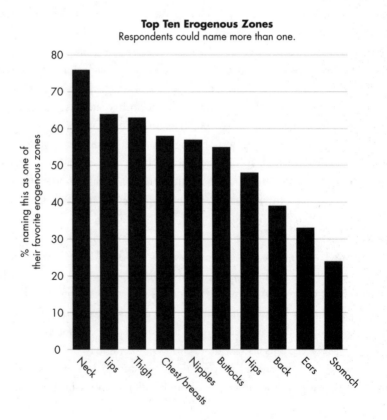

Top Ten Erogenous Zones
Respondents could name more than one.

I ♥ ORGASMS

And don't forget these other fave spots named by survey respondents: shoulders, hands/wrists, feet, back of knees, waist, head, and lower torso just above the pubic hair. The truth is, *any* body part can be an erogenous zone if it's touched in the right way by the right partner at the right time. A small percentage of people can have orgasms from having their breasts or other parts of their body stroked without any below-the-waist genital stimulation.

In some cases, the overall percentages don't tell the full story. For example, neck was the top pick for most respondents, including cis men and women, and trans people overall. But looking more closely at the data, buttocks was the top pick for trans feminine respondents who weren't taking hormones. For trans feminine folks taking hormones, breasts perked up into first place, as opposed to trans masculine folks, for whom breasts didn't even make the top ten.

Bottom line: The zone that makes one person shiver with delight might make the next one's skin crawl or trigger feelings of dysphoria. Asking for what you like, and tuning into your partner's cues and requests, will let you unlock the thrill of erogenous zone power boosts.

Multiple Orgasms: Double Dipping Is Allowed!

AFTER THEIR BIG O, some clitoris-owners find it easy to continue and have two or more orgasms before their arousal fades away. Others have a single orgasm and find their clitoris gets too sensitive to have any more stimulation, just as most people don't want their penis touched after they come. That's perfectly fine. Orgasms aren't like trading cards: the more you collect, the better. A person with a vulva can be deeply fulfilled and sexually thrilled with only one orgasm per sexual interlude (or even none at all).

That said, if you have a vulva and you're curious about having multiple orgasms but haven't been able to, try this tip from Betty Dodson, author of *Sex for One* and *Orgasms for Two*: After one orgasm, stop the clitoral stimulation for a short period of time, like ten seconds or a minute. Then, try resuming clitoral stimulation. For

Same Concept, Multiplied

IN JAPANESE, THE word for masturbation with a penis is *senzuri*, which means "one thousand strokes." The word for masturbation for a person with a clitoris? *Manzuri*: "ten thousand strokes."

most people, the period of hypersensitivity passes quite quickly, and then they can start toward another orgasm (or several more, with a short break in between each one). For some, each orgasm in a string gets bigger and bigger; for others, they get smaller and smaller. Even in a series of multiple orgasms, each climax requires its own buildup (different than little "aftershocks" that are part of the original orgasm).

Although penis-owners are capable of multiple orgasms (see the box on page 39), multiples tend to come far more easily to those with a vulva. This is at least in part because, though all genitals have erectile tissue that swells with blood during arousal, the blood can flow in and out of vulvas and clitorises faster and more easily, so those parts can "refill" and "reorgasm" repeatedly.

Kegel Your Way to Bigger, Better Orgasms

BACK IN THE 1950s, a gynecologist named Dr. Arnold Kegel invented exercises that helped his patients with urinary incontinence by strengthening the muscles surrounding the vagina and urethra. As the patients' muscle tone improved, they discovered a lovely side effect to the exercises: better orgasms! Dr. Kegel's good name would never have been remembered so fondly if his exercises had merely resulted in better bladder control.

Further research has found that indeed, learning both how to strengthen and relax the pubococcygeus muscle group (conveniently called the PC muscles, since "pubococcygeus" sounds more like a rare disease than a sexy group of muscles) increases blood flow to the pelvic area, increases sensitivity, and sometimes results in stronger orgasms for people of all genders. Many people with a penis say they enjoy it if their partner's PC muscles are toned enough to squeeze their penis during vaginal sex.

Some people have an unconscious habit of keeping their PC muscles tight (*hypertonic* is the technical term) all the time, the same way some people clench their jaws or forget to relax their shoulders. This causes just as many problems as weak muscles, including pain during penetration and burning, aching, numbness, or itching of the genitals. Diagnoses like vaginismus and vulvodynia can all be related to overly tense pelvic floor muscles, and in this case, doing Kegel squeezes (without the "relaxes") can actually make matters worse. Practicing relaxing these muscles is a key part of Kegel success. Pelvic floor therapists can be a huge help in diagnosing and treating these types of issues.

> *Kegels are amazing!!! They make orgasms much more of an experience that you can actually FEEL.*

> *I was diagnosed with a hypertonic pelvic floor. Kegels will put my pelvic floor into spasm so I can't do them, but I've worked hard to strengthen my core and learn to relax.*

> *I have been trying to do "the squeeze" more while in the act of sexual intercourse and have found it to improve both my boyfriend's and my own pleasure a lot!*

Five Reasons That Kegels Rock

(at least for some people)

1. You don't have to buy any special equipment that will take up half your apartment.
2. You can do them in any position, including standing in line, sitting in front of your computer, lying in bed, and practicing headstands.
3. Because no one can tell you're doing them, you can get in shape while carrying on a conversation with your professor, boss, or Great-Aunt Sue.
4. You can multitask, transforming annoying waits in the supermarket checkout line, while your Wi-Fi is lagging, and on hold (what purpose does hold music have beyond providing a beat for one's sexercise?).
5. How many other exercises might actually improve your sex life?

Dorian's Kegel Tip

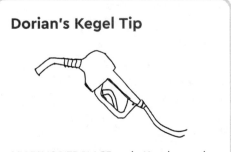

MY FAVORITE PLACE to do Kegels is at the gas pump. The best ones for this purpose make a steady click, click, clicking sound while you fill 'er up. I discovered that since there's nothing else to do while I wait, the clicks are a great way to work out my PC muscles. I can challenge myself to hold for a full ten clicks, relax fully, then do quick squeeze-relax-squeeze in rhythm with the clicks, even trying double-time squeezes. As long as you maintain the same bored expression on your face as everyone else at the gas station, no one will have any clue what you're up to. When you really get into it, you'll find you're disappointed when the pump clicks off, signaling a full gas tank and the end to your workout.

To do Kegel exercises, identify the muscles you're going to be working out. They're the same muscles you use if you're peeing and want to stop the flow of urine. In general, you should do the exercises when you're *not* peeing—which, lucky for you, is most of the day—but when you're just starting out, try squeezing your PC muscles while you pee at least once to make sure you've identified the right muscles.

There are two different kinds of exercises you can practice:

Long squeezes. Pull in as if you were squeezing a finger with equal pressure on all sides. Count to three, then fully relax the muscles. Repeat. Remember that the "fully relax" part of Kegels is as important as the squeezing. As the muscles get stronger, hold the count to higher numbers before relaxing all the way. Can you reach ten? Twenty? Keep breathing while you squeeze. Some people like to imagine they are pulling an elevator up inside their body.

Fast little squeezes. Squeeze the muscles in short pulses as if you were following the beat to a song. It's hard to do very fast beats at first, but as you get stronger, you'll be able to pulse faster. Remember to let the muscles relax after each beat. Don't forget to keep breathing!

Try to remember to do the exercises for at least a few minutes every day, increasing the number of repetitions or the length of the holds as you feel yourself gain strength. Some people find it feels sort of "yucky" at first to work out these muscles, just as it can feel unpleasant to work any muscle that's out of shape. Continue trying to do small numbers of Kegels, and you'll find you get stronger quite quickly. Keeping these muscles in good shape throughout your life is good for vaginal and urinary health (yes, the doctor may have

Are You Coming, Going, or Enjoying?

RESEARCHERS AT NATIONAL Taiwan University asked native speakers of twenty-seven languages about the phrases and expressions related to orgasm in their languages. One of their more fascinating sets of results was what phrase one might say to announce one is about to have—or in the process of having—an orgasm.

Nearly half the languages studied use some version of the "I'm coming" that's familiar to English speakers. These include *Geliyourum* (I am coming) in Turkish, *sto venendo* (I come) in Italian, and *Ateinu tuojau tuojau* (I'm coming right away/immediately) in Lithuanian.

Several languages, including Japanese and Portuguese, use a phrase along the lines of "I'm going," and several more, including Russian, have a version of "I'm ending/finishing." The researchers asked their Japanese participants if having an orgasm means "going," where are you going, exactly? "According to the Japanese speakers in the study, the usage of *Iku* ('[I'm] going') in Japanese actually implies death and the process of ascending to heaven," they write. French, too, references death in their language's phrase for orgasm, *la petite mort* (the little death).

Other announcements of the moment of orgasm include *nyt mä tulen* (now I'm [the] fire) in Finnish, *Eu estou gozando* (I'm enjoying) in Brazilian Portuguese, and *Už budu* ([I] will be) in Czech. That last puzzled the researchers, but Czech interviewees pointed out that the concept is fairly similar to René Descartes's famous line "I think, therefore, I am." Czech speakers described the phrase as suggesting that orgasm is about the process of being, the state of being alive.

We'd put it this way: "I'm about to orgasm, therefore I am." Descartes was on to something!

> **Fun Fact**
>
> IF HUMANS HAD tails, you'd use your PC muscles, the same ones you use to do Kegel exercises, to wag your tail.

prescribed Kegels to your grandmother), as well as preparing for and getting back in shape after childbirth. That said, be cautious not to overdo Kegels if you suspect that your issue may be too much pelvic floor tension. If fully relaxing is tough for you, get thee to a pelvic floor therapist!

Because the biggest challenge to this exercise routine is remembering to do it, it helps to find some regular occurrence that's your "cue" to Kegel—ideally, something you do most days like wait for the subway, ride an elevator, or the most classic cue of all, sit in the car at a red light. (We think it would be a helpful reminder if the word "KEGEL!" were imprinted on every red light as a reminder.)

I do Kegels sometimes, when I remember to do them or when I'm nervous and fidgety and I'm trying to avoid cracking my knuckles.

Fantasy: Imagination for Grown-Ups

OUR SURVEY FOUND that 35 percent of people with a vulva fantasize at least some of the time while they're being sexual with a partner, and 79 percent do so when they're masturbating. Fantasizing is tapping into the power of whatever images or stories turn you on and help you reach those highest levels of arousal that launch orgasms. There's nothing shameful about allowing yourself to put these images to use: most people of all genders do! Because the mind is the biggest sex organ, as you've probably heard, it's perfectly logical that you'd want to use yours to help you come. The movies you watch in your mind are private. No one ever has to know what they are unless you choose to share them.

Multiple Orgasms—for Penises?

VULVA-OWNERS AREN'T THE only ones with the capacity to be multi-orgasmic. Penises can have more than one orgasm too. The capability comes naturally to some preadolescents and young adults, but it's also possible for older people to learn—with a considerable amount of work. The main part of the penis-owner's workout involves doing lots and lots of Kegel exercises, described on pages 34–36, 38. You likely already have enough strength in your PC muscles to stop yourself from peeing midstream. For most people with a penis, orgasm and ejaculation happen at the same time, but Kegels can help you build up enough strength in that muscle to be able to experience orgasm without ejaculation. After a steady Kegel workout for at least several months, when you're at the point when you're about to ejaculate, you may be able to clamp down on the PC muscle and have the intense, pleasurable sensations of an orgasm while preventing yourself from ejaculating. Because you haven't ejaculated, you can do this over and over again to be multiorgasmic. For those interested in pursuing this, a small industry of books and websites instruct in more detail how to use this and other techniques for penis-owners to become multiorgasmic.

Sexual fantasies are what keeps me in the mood most of the time. It's so easy for me to stop being aroused. If I wish to continue, it's almost pivotal for me to fantasize.

The most important thing I learned that helped me have orgasms was to be unashamed of my fantasies, even if they are sometimes socially taboo, and to be honest about sharing them with my partner. That freed my mind up quite a bit to really enjoy coming.

Fantasies don't help me. I've tried to use this technique, but it doesn't do it for me. I think I rely more on physical stimulation on my entire body than on images in my head or what I'm looking at in reality.

Video-Based Orgasm Education

OMGYES.COM IS AN online collection of hundreds of educational videos (not porn) intended to teach very specific ways that some vulva-owners like to be pleasured. Their content uses clothes-off videos, interviews, and animations to let you see the techniques they're teaching in detail. You pay a one-time fee to buy each collection of dozens of videos. They say they're working on new video collections about pleasure for penis-owners, transgender pleasure, and pleasure in menopause and after childbirth—maybe those have already been released as you read this. Several of our survey respondents said it was helpful in learning how to have an orgasm. We think it's a treasure map you'll want to know about.

As a young teenager, Dorian had heard about fantasizing and, lying in bed one night, decided she'd try it. She imagined a huge bed and spent some time mentally decorating the bedroom, imagining the silky sheets and luscious comforter. She pictured herself naked in the bed. (That's how sex happens, right?) Then, she thought, *I need a man*. (She hadn't yet named or admitted her same-sex attractions.) Searching her memory banks for a sexy image of a man, what came to mind was a character who resembled all the princes in Disney movies: broad shoulders, chiseled jaw, sparkling smile. She imagined her personal Disney prince walking over to the bed, and then the fantasy stalled. She didn't know what she wanted to have happen next, and she wasn't feeling turned on *at all*. Of course not: it wasn't a real sexual fantasy, just a weird fusion of too many Disney cartoons and interior design catalogs.

Some people know exactly what fantasies turn them on or might replay the memory of a favorite sexual interlude or a movie scene that made them wet (or hard). If you're coming up empty-handed in your search for fantasies, one easy source of ideas is erotica, stories written to arouse. For this purpose, we recommend stories rather than pictures or videos because they engage your imagination and allow you to create your own mental images. There are fantastic books of erotica, but if you're trying to figure out what you like, nothing is faster and easier than exploring free erotica sites online. These have thousands of stories divided into categories, some predictable and others you wouldn't imagine in your wildest dreams. Skimming a few in each category can be fascinating because some will summon your inner "ick!" while others will intrigue you. Take note of those stories that get your blood flowing, the ones that really absorb you. Soon, you'll get a sense of what genres you like and which details grab you. When you're being sexual later, replay them in your mind, using your own imagination to tweak the plot or improve the characters. Before long, you'll be fantasizing like a champion!

I watch or read sex stories, then fantasize about my sex partner doing those things to me. It's helped me figure out what I like and don't like.

I figured out my fantasies by hearing about different fantasies of other people, and whichever turned me on the most and sounded like something I would try became a fantasy of my own. I may have modified them a bit, because of what I already know I do and don't like.

I figured out what I liked from pornography, and I often play one particular scene in my head when I'm with or without a partner.

I knew I was queer when my sex dreams and fantasies included all genders. The main focus is usually on breasts and nipples.

Many trans and nonbinary people find fantasy can be super affirming as well as arousing. In a fantasy, bodies can look, feel, and function however you want them to.

My fantasy life changed after I came out. I felt more free to fantasize about myself with different anatomy.

In my dreams it feels like a perfect world. I don't have boobs, and my clitoris works like a cock. I'm just a person, and everything is normal and everyone is satisfied. I need to figure out how to translate this into real life.

Fantasies that turn you on may be things you'd like to act out someday, especially if the situation were right and you had a partner you particularly trusted. Other fantasies that get you going may involve situations your analytic mind finds downright problematic or offensive, that you never, ever want to have happen in the real world. For example, numerous studies find it's quite common for people to fantasize about being overpowered and forced to have sex; some research even finds it's among the most common sexual fantasies for women.

Prioritizing Consent

AT ITS SIMPLEST, consent means agreeing about what you're going to do together. In partnered sexual encounters, consent is more than just agreeing to have sex—it also means you agree about what types of sex you'll have, and where and how you'll touch and be touched. Throughout this book, we'll highlight ways you can check in and get consent as things heat up, but for now, remember: sex without consent is sexual assault. For more on consent, see page 259.

Obviously, it can be disturbing to be aroused by a rape scenario, particularly if one is horrified by the idea of rape in real life. Many researchers and those who enjoy these fantasies point out that a sexual fantasy is definitely *not* the same thing as a sexual desire. Just because you find it sexy to imagine a given scene does *not* mean you ever want this scene to come true. In fact, there are huge differences: In a fantasy (even a fantasy of being forced to do something), the person fantasizing is actually in total control. You create the imaginary situation and decide exactly what will happen and when it will end. Exactly the opposite is true in a real-world rape, where the victim is powerless and is definitely not controlling what happens to them. Many people say understanding this difference has helped them both sort out the confusing feelings that can arise if these are the fantasies that turn them on and give themselves permission to use the fantasies that work for them.

Of course, if you're concerned that you may act on a fantasy that could be dangerous to yourself or others, it may be wise to turn your imagination down a different path. You can seek professional help if that's too hard to do on your own.

The universe of sexual fantasies is limitless. Here are just a few examples that vulva-owners shared in our survey:

ACCORDING TO THE Kinsey and Hite reports, 1 to 2 percent of women can have an orgasm from fantasy alone, with no genital stimulation at all. Lucky!

I fantasize about being with my partner. He turns me on so much, I just think about the times we've been together. Sometimes I throw Brad Pitt in it, too.

I fantasize about women touching me instead of my male partner.

If I fantasize about being an exotic dancer, I can dress and act accordingly, which I've found to improve my libido and hunger for sex. It may be the excitement of trying something new or putting away conventional and shameful beliefs about having sex that allows me to enjoy it more. I feel as though if I'm someone else, I can shamelessly flaunt my passion and desire for sex.

I usually think about a penis inside of me (especially my partner's) and not just during masturbation. I think about it even while the penis is inside of me. I think it just turns me on so much quicker. I don't know why; it just works for me. I don't have any other image. I just solely focus on the penis.

I consider myself straight, but I almost always fantasize about women going down on me. I just find women's bodies so hot! I want to be in a long-term relationship with a man, but women are beautiful and exciting as well. It could also be that I've never hooked up with a girl before, which makes it even more forbidden and exciting.

One of the things that I fantasize about (which is difficult for me as a feminist, especially a sex-positive feminist) is rape. Sometimes I find it incredibly arousing. I'm almost certain it's the power thing that turns me on. In my fantasies I see the survivor/victim (which is usually me) as powerful because of my sexual prowess, and the rapist as completely unable to control himself. I know that this is nothing like rape in real life, and when I think about actually being raped I'm completely terrified.

Many people who fantasize while they masturbate aren't sure about the etiquette of doing so while they're with a partner. We believe that doing so is fine, quite common, and another way to increase the likelihood of an orgasm. Because fantasizing happens only inside your own head, it's not cheating, as some worry, but harnessing the erotic power of your mind. (Those of us who grew up with the cultural baggage that "women should be polite" and keep our thoughts lovingly on our partner at all times should remember, too, that many partners who didn't grow up with that baggage fantasize during every sexual encounter, keep their thoughts private, and never think twice about it.) The best kinds of fantasies during partnered sex are often blended, where you mentally integrate your partner's caresses, strength, or softness into the story, so the real-life sex and fantasy sex merge. It's up to you whether you choose to share the fact that you were fantasizing, or the details, with your partner. Talking about or acting out a fantasy with a partner you trust can build intimacy—not to mention being totally sexy. In fact, the powerhouse combination of fantasy and masturbation is why some people—especially those in long-distance relationships—swear by sexting and FaceTime sex.

My boyfriend is away a lot, so I have to imagine what I would be doing with him. That usually leads to more than just imagining. Also, we'll talk about our fantasies together and that will give us ideas of what to do or even cause us to both want to jump on each other right then.

My girlfriend and I are aware that we each fantasize during sex. We talk each other through scenarios. They help me orgasm. I've always had difficulty orgasming from pure physical stimulation.

I have had success in the past writing out fantasies or telling a partner one as a bedtime story, step-by-step. Then letting them know I'd like to do that.

Clitoral Tips for Partners

IF YOUR PARTNER has a clitoris, just locating it and rubbing merrily away as if you've found Aladdin's lamp isn't going to do the trick. Whether you're using your fingers, your tongue, a vibrator, or something else, here are a few tips:

○ **Don't reach for the clit too early in the sexual interaction.** Most clit-owners find it likes to be touched only after they're already somewhat aroused.
○ **Start with indirect touch.** A person with a clitoris may love to be touched very gently through their pants or underwear before they're ready for more direct stimulation.

> *Try touching around the area or put a clothing article between your hand and her body (silk scarves are VERY effective).*

○ **Be gentle.** Once your partner is ready for skin-to-skin touch, touch and stroke their outer vaginal lips with a light touch. Slowly work your way inside. Once you're touching the clitoris, remember, this is an exquisitely sensitive organ. Being "gentle" and "soft" were the most common pieces of advice clitoris-owners in our survey gave partners about how to touch their genitals. You can start at the top of the shaft, just under the bone, and move down closer to the head if they want you to. Your partner may want firmer pressure, but ask about that or follow the clit-owner's lead. ("More, harder!" is a much better response than "Ow!")

○ **Keep it wet.** For any touch that's inside the outer labia, lick your fingers, add lube, or dip into the vagina's wetness to wet and rewet the clit. Dry touching doesn't feel good to most clitoris-owners.

○ **Give and get feedback.** Sometimes, it can be helpful to break down clitoral touching into three key components: *directness, pressure*, and *speed*. These can be helpful for couple communication, whether you're the one asking for feedback or the one giving directions. You can check in about whether your partner wants their clitoris touched right on the tip versus the shaft or farther away (directness), how hard they want the stimulation to be (pressure), and how fast they want the movement to be (speed).

○ **Use hands and eyes.** Invite your partner to move your hand where they want it, or rest your hand over theirs so you can get the hang of the movements they like. If your sweetie will let you watch them masturbate, that's a great way to see how they like to be touched.

> *I've watched my partner masturbate—it was very helpful to me. It allowed me to see which part of her vaginal area she touched the most and how she touched it. It allowed me to see how many fingers she likes inside of her. Really watching her do it was a turn-on as well as an educational experience. And after watching, I could imitate the things she did to herself and she knew I had paid attention. (And there's nothing women like more than knowing someone is paying attention to them, right?)*

○ **Stimulate multiple parts at once.** Many people with a clitoris love having other parts of their body touched simultaneously with clitoral stimulation. (But be warned: actually pulling this off can be a bit like rubbing your head and patting your stomach at the same time.)

○ **Ask, ask, ask.** What any individual likes varies *dramatically*. It varies person to person. Even for the same person it could be different at different points in their menstrual cycle. It changes as you age. Ask your partner to guide you and teach you, and be open to learning the nuances of their body's dance. If you don't know what to say, ask, "How's this?" or short questions like "Up here?" "Side to side like this?" "Harder?" Don't expect your partner to read your mind. Appreciate their efforts, make adjustments, give gentle suggestions, and provide plenty of positive feedback about what works!

Every woman is different, so ask what she likes. Some don't like it right on the clitoris, some do, but either way, don't rub it like you're trying to sandpaper something down. It hurts after a while. Penetration is good too, but don't go too deep. Realize that the canal curves. Some partners wave their fingers around in there and it just feels weird, like there is a fish out of water up your vagina. Just rub around a little and massage the inside slowly.

As an autistic person, receiving physical touch is very overwhelming to my senses. My clitoris is especially sensitive, and the head is like a nuke button. I would prefer if people didn't assume the ways in which it is okay to touch me even after it's been established that I have the desire to have sex with them.

Sweet Dreams

BETWEEN 6 AND 37 percent of people with a vulva report having had orgasms in their sleep, depending on the study.

In my sleep I get vaginal orgasms, which I can't achieve through sex, and I like those the best. My vaginal muscles start tightening and spasming, and I wake up and it just feels really good.

- ○ **Enjoy yourself.** It can be hard to relax and enjoy if one gets the sense that one's partner is bored, uncomfortable, or disinterested. On the flip side, if your partner is clearly enjoying themselves (or even turned on), that's fun! Don't let clit play become a chore; it'll stop working.
- ○ **Stick with it.** Once the object of your affection is close to coming, don't change what you're doing. This is not the time to add variety or mix things up! Stay in the same spot, doing the same movement, until they come or instruct you otherwise.

For Those Who Have Experienced Abuse or Assault

[Content note: The following section includes some personal quotes and stories about abuse and assault.]

Traumatic sexual experiences, like sexual abuse or sexual assault, can have a long-lasting impact on one's sexuality. This is true regardless of exactly what happened, whatever your gender, whether the events were one time or repeated, whether they happened as a child or an adult, and whether they were perpetrated by a stranger, relative, partner, friend, doctor, teacher, or someone else. If you're a survivor of abuse or assault, you could face a myriad of different sexual challenges, including:

- Difficulty getting aroused or having orgasms
- Emotions, memories, or flashbacks of the traumatic event(s) related to certain kinds of touch or positions
- Guilt about enjoying sex
- Lack of interest in sex
- Having sex compulsively even when you know it's physically or emotionally unhealthy or unsafe
- Discomfort with what kind of sex you like or what fantasies turn you on
- Dissociating: keeping yourself mentally or emotionally separate from what you're experiencing physically during sex

Sadly, given how common sexual abuse and sexual assault are, these issues and others affect too large a percentage of people.

I was assaulted by a boyfriend when I was seventeen, and it has definitely affected the way I experience sexual relationships and pleasure. I sometimes don't orgasm because I flash back to the assault and freeze up.

I haven't orgasmed in over a decade because of sexual trauma.

On the subject of orgasm, some survivors are confused because they had an orgasm while they were being abused or assaulted, or found the experience physically pleasurable. This does not mean that they wanted the abuse: physical arousal, pleasure, and orgasm are the body's automatic, physiological responses to certain kinds of stimulation. Even if a survivor experienced these things, the experience was still unwanted and abusive.

I was raped when I was eleven. I'm just now able to begin to heal. As a survivor, I numbed myself from anything sexual. I dissociated my mind from my body. I still have trouble with masturbation—I have trouble not having flashbacks when I do it. I also have trouble feeling any kind of pleasure because when I was raped I did feel pleasure. I can't get past my mental blocks yet, but I WILL!

The good news: It *is* possible to have a healthy, positive sex life after experiencing sexual trauma. The journey may (or may not) involve therapy, helpful books and websites, a support group, introspection, journaling, and a supportive partner.

I was date-raped when I was eighteen years old. Sometimes I think about that when I'm having sex and start sobbing and can't continue with the sex. Now I am taking some "time off" to learn how to have a healthy sexuality, starting with myself.

I was raped in high school, and for the next five years it affected both sexual experiences and the way I treated myself. The majority of my lovers were wonderful, warm, generous people, so it was time that healed my wounds, and now I respect my body and have the best sex life I could ever hope for.

For many who have experienced sexual trauma, sharing what they've learned about their sexual needs and limits helps improve partnered sex tremendously.

I'm a survivor of sexual assault so this is a super important conversation I have every time. It's really awkward but you just kinda gotta do it, and the way better sex you get out of it is a great incentive to keep going.

For Support and Healing

RAPE, ABUSE, AND Incest National Network
www.rainn.org
National hotline, live chat support, and tons of great articles & info

FORGE
www.forge-forward.org
Resources for transgender and nonbinary sexual violence survivors and
   their partners

1 IN 6
www.1in6.org
Chat-based support groups and resources for men who have experienced
   sexual abuse or assault

There have been many times where we just had to stop altogether. Sometimes it's not even that my partner did anything wrong; it's just the headspace I'm in at the time that won't let me let go of the past.

Partners and allies can join survivors in working to end sexual violence. Some choose to get involved as volunteers at their local rape crisis center, or to participate in a campus or community group that educates about sexual violence prevention. National groups like Men Can Stop Rape (www.mcsr.org) and the National Sexual Violence Resource Center (www.nsvrc.org) provide trainings and educational materials.

All people have the right to reclaim their sexual lives and find healthy, fulfilling, consensual sensuality and sexuality. The essential work continues as survivors, partners of survivors, and allies of all genders join together to create a culture free of sexual violence.

If Experiencing Pleasure Is a Challenge

LOTS OF THINGS affect our ability to experience pleasure and orgasms. We really like Emily Nagoski's metaphor in her excellent book *Come as You Are*. She says, imagine we're each given a little plot of fertile land at birth, a garden that represents our future sexual selves. When we're young, our family and our culture plant things there for us and tend the garden. Maybe they plant messages of acceptance and confidence, or maybe they sow seeds of shame and insecurity. As we get older, we start to learn how to care for our garden, beginning by looking around at what's growing there and how best to care for our sexual selves. By adulthood, they hand the whole thing over to us.

Some of us reach adulthood and realize our "garden" is full of toxic plants that we may choose slowly to weed out: destructive messages from parents, religious communities, or friends; poor information about caring for our body; dishonest advice about relationships. Some of us feel as if we were handed a lush, fertile garden that just needs a bit of pruning as we find our way to our authentic adult sexual selves.

> *I grew up in a religious and conservative (Catholic) household that would shame any sexual encounter outside a hetero marriage. This hindered a lot of my exploration into my own sexuality until I was in my early- to mid-twenties. I feel like I lost out on a lot of figuring out who I am based on religious shame and guilt which I've moved on from.*

Survivors of sexual trauma may find that experience contaminated their soil, making it tough for healthy plants to grow. With time and patient fertilization, it's absolutely possible to enrich that soil and cultivate a thriving garden.

But trauma survivors aren't the only ones who may find that the "garden" they've inherited is making it tough to experience sexual pleasure. It's never too late to take a look around your own little plot of land and think about what's been planted there by parents, relatives, teachers, faith traditions, and culture. If you suspect some of what you find there is getting in the way of your ability to experience pleasure in your body, you have the power to weed it out and identify new values and messages that will make space for your own sexual pleasure to flower.

Some First Orgasm Stories

WE TREASURE THE thousands of stories vulva-owners have shared with us about their first time having a big O. Here are some of our favorites.

I had seen those TV commercials that showed women shampooing their hair in a tropical waterfall. It looked so sexy! One day when I was ten or twelve I acted it out in the shower. I imagined the tropical fruit and the waterfall. As I soaped up my body, I imagined a man in the bushes watching me. As the water ran over me, I rubbed myself between my legs—and I had my first orgasm.

I was a freshman in high school, and I was at a sleepover party with a bunch of friends. Someone had a magazine with an article about how to masturbate. We were all like "Let's try it!" There were a lot of first orgasms that night.

I think my first orgasm was as a young teen in the bath rubbing my body against full water balloons. I was pretending they were my penis and then realized that they felt really good against my vulva.

As a little kid, I was an avid humper. Pillows, stuffed animals, the floor. I can't remember the first time I orgasmed, but I remember the amazing feeling of it and that I wanted to do it all the time. Some of my earliest memories are of my parents yelling at me to stop humping things!

Several people, and one mother of a toddler daughter, have told us they (or their daughter) had this experience:

When I was a little kid I was riding in the car with my parents. I was sitting in the back seat in a car seat—I don't know how old I was, but I was little enough that I still rode in a car seat. The car seat had this plastic safety bar that ran between my legs, and one day I discovered that if I squirmed against the bar it felt really good. I was a really happy little kid on long car rides.

When I was nineteen, I had my first boyfriend. After we'd been dating for a while, masturbation came up in conversation, and I told him I had never masturbated. He was totally horrified—he had trouble believing me, but I convinced him I was telling the truth. He said, "I'm going to give you a lesson." He sat me down and taught me how to masturbate. I had my first orgasm then and there!

At least three different people have separately told us experiences nearly identical to this one:

I was in high school, and this was when they had the Presidential Physical Fitness Program [which required that all public school students practice and compete at certain exercises]. I was doing that exercise where you pull yourself into a chin-up and hold it as long as you can. And while I held myself in this chin-up I had my first orgasm. At first I didn't know what was happening, but it was incredible.

Apparently when President Kennedy instituted this national physical fitness program for schoolchildren (a version of which still exists today), he had no idea how many first orgasms he would facilitate. We've heard similar stories of kids and adults having these kinds of climaxes, sometimes called "coregasms," from having all their muscles tensed, vaginas included, while doing sit-ups or doing leg lifts using a gym's weight machine. Most of us aren't able to come this way, but those who can have extra incentive to stay in shape!

When I was a little kid I had a Raggedy Ann doll I used to rub against and have orgasms. I remember one day I asked my mom if what I was doing was okay, and she said, "Of course, dear, it's perfectly normal. You go right on dancing with Raggedy Ann."

The first time I got close to having an orgasm my heart was pounding so hard I was worried that I was going to have a heart attack or something, so I almost stopped. After a while I decided that maybe I didn't care and I should just go ahead. Turned out it wasn't a heart attack.

My first orgasm happened accidentally in the pool. I moved against the jet that shoots from the side of the pool underwater, and got a really great feeling. So I stayed there until I got a rolling feeling in my stomach and my privates started throbbing. I didn't really think about what it meant, I just liked the feeling. I did that every summer.

In college I've had a few male friends who used to constantly pester me about whether I masturbated. I would always say no, which was true, but they didn't believe me and they were always badgering me about it. It was a topic of conversation a lot. One day it was winter break and I was finally alone. There weren't a lot of people on campus and I didn't have much to do, so I thought, I'll try it. I did—and I had an orgasm. It was great. [I] called my guy friends, and said, "I tried it, and it worked!" I was thrilled.

Sometimes the nudge that leads to a first orgasm is related to words and mental space rather than a change in physical stimulation.

I came out as trans to my now-ex-boyfriend. The next time we got rowdy together, he made sure to address me with male diminutives, and that was the final push. We later broke up because he wasn't entirely comfortable, but I am thankful for the acceptance and validation he yielded to me in that moment— and the orgasm it caused!

And sometimes it's a combination of affirmation and physical stimulation:

I would say my first gender-affirming orgasm had to be on my own with my Satisfyer vibe. It was my first vibrator ever, and the shape of it allows me to put my Tdick in the hole. All I did was grind against it, but it was incredibly validating and felt amazing.

2

So, You Want to Have an Orgasm?

You've never had an orgasm, but you want to? Not sure whether you've had a big O? You've come to the right place! (If you and/or your partner already have orgasms, and you're happy with them, you might want to skip to the next chapter.) More people with a vulva haven't had orgasms than you might think: About half of us have our first orgasm after age sixteen. It's *very* common for clit-owners not to learn how to come until they're in college or in their twenties. And the learning curve continues well beyond that: we've met plenty who had their first orgasm in their thirties, forties, and beyond. This chapter may also be useful for those who find it's more challenging to reach those lightning bolts of orgasm than they'd like, and for supportive partners trying to help.

This chapter is focused on the needs of people with a vulva and clitoris having their first orgasm. Our transgender and nonbinary readers who have those body parts may find useful information in this chapter and also in Chapter 9.

Not Sure

IN OUR SURVEY, 7 percent of cisgender women said they didn't know whether they'd had an orgasm. Some ask their friends for help figuring out whether they have or not and often get a response along the lines of "If you'd had one, you'd know." So unhelpful! Our work, and our conversations with others like pleasure activist Betty Dodson who helped countless women have their first orgasm, leads us to believe there are two possible explanations for why so many people aren't sure if they've come:

1. They've felt intense pleasure but not an orgasm. They feel unclear because typical arousal involves surges of pleasure, sometimes quite intense. These surges are usually shorter than orgasms, may not have the same kind of full-body involvement as an orgasm, and while they feel good, aren't *as* good as an orgasm. But how could you know that unless you've had both?

2. They've been having small orgasms. Sometimes people see porn orgasms, or read descriptions of orgasms, and imagine the experience to be much bigger and more earth-shattering than the little orgasms they're experiencing. They know they're feeling *something*, but they're not convinced it's an orgasm. Pleasure-seekers in this situation may be able to "grow" their orgasms with Kegel exercises or by building up to higher levels of arousal before they allow themselves to come. Or they may begin to appreciate what they have, and recognize that porn-gasms are like porn star breasts: bigger—and faker—than most of what you'll find in the real world.

I think I had a very definite impression of what orgasm was supposed to be and put pressure on myself to embody that image. Then I ran across an online article that emphasized that orgasm can take many different forms. I also finally internalized the idea that orgasm is not the end goal, and that as long as I feel satisfied by my sexual interactions (with or without orgasm), I shouldn't feel disappointed. Incidentally, since then it's been much easier to orgasm.

What If I'm One of Those People Who Can't Have Orgasms?

MANY PEOPLE HAVE heard the distressing claim, "Some people just can't have orgasms." As a result, those who've never had one sometimes worry that they might be one of the unfortunate ones. Although many studies have found that 5 to 10 percent of women have never had an orgasm, this statistic is misleading. Many of these nonorgasmers are young and haven't learned how to have an orgasm *yet*. In the classic *Hite Report*, the majority of women who'd never had an orgasm were thirty or younger—which suggests that even those who didn't used to be orgasmic often figure out how to come as they get older.

I had three children before I ever had an orgasm. I was married, and we had a good sex life—I enjoyed sex a lot. It wasn't until years later that I realized just how good it could get.

Viagra for Vulvas?

SOME FRUSTRATED VULVA-OWNERS muse about how nice it would be just to pop a pill for instant orgasms. Some find Viagra, Cialis, or similar drugs tempting. Unfortunately, research studies have conclusively found that Viagra and its competitor pharmaceuticals don't work for people with a vulva. Although Viagra increases blood flow to the vagina and clitoris (as it does for a penis), this doesn't result in higher levels of arousal. Some people with a vulva who took Viagra in clinical trials did have more orgasms—the rate was the same for vulva-owners who were being given sugar pills they believed were Viagra. The placebo effect is powerful!

Viagra and all the others have very real medical risks and side effects. Although some doctors still prescribe them to their patients with a vulva, there's no evidence that they're worth taking.

Also included in that 5 to 10 percent who have never had an orgasm are those who are too uncomfortable to read a book like this one, experiment with masturbating, buy a vibrator, or take any of the other steps that are most likely to lead to them becoming orgasmic. Some may be perfectly satisfied not having orgasms, and see no reason to pursue the matter. The percentage of people with a clitoris who would like to have an orgasm but are truly physically unable to is minuscule. Statistically speaking, it's highly unlikely that you're one of them.

For a long period of time, I was unable to have orgasms, even though I'd been able to have them before. I think much of the problem was psychological, in that I worried something might be wrong with me. I was more anxious about having an orgasm, and so it became harder and harder to relax when I did want to masturbate or have sex. It's very easy to get yourself into a self-fulfilling prophecy like "I can't have an orgasm!" Then you try to masturbate or have sex, and don't come, which reaffirms that you can't have an orgasm. After many months of no orgasms at all, I found myself in a very low-pressure situation with a willing and eager partner, and I was able to have orgasms again.

Five Steps to Your First Orgasm

READY TO GIVE it a try? You can do these activities at your own pace, definitely not all in one day. It'll probably take at least a few weeks, and possibly a few months or longer, to work your way through them, depending on how often you work on it.

Step One: Start Alone

Most people in relationships have already done things that could lead to orgasm: touching the clitoris, using fingers to stimulate the G-spot, oral sex, and possibly intercourse in various positions. If these haven't already led to orgasm, and you're ready to take on having an orgasm as an official project, it may be tempting to make it a joint one. Our best advice is to resist this temptation. That doesn't mean you can't have sex with your partner during the time you're learning how to have an orgasm—just don't make having an orgasm the focus of your time together.

Unlikely Orgasms

A SMALL BODY of research finds that many vulva-owners are able to have orgasms even after accidents or surgeries that might have been assumed to make this impossible. For instance, many whose clitoris has been partly or entirely removed during female circumcision (also called female genital mutilation) still have orgasms, some reporting that their breasts became their most sexually arousing organ. Similarly, up to half of those with spinal cord injuries, whose body doesn't transmit nerve impulses from below their injury, are able to experience and enjoy orgasms from genital stimulation, even though they can't feel the touch that brings it on. Although experts once told spinal cord injury survivors that the orgasms they claimed to experience were "all in your head" and "not real," laboratory researchers have now confirmed that these orgasms are as physiologically real as anyone else's.

Rather than thinking about yourself as nonorgasmic, it's helpful to think of yourself as preorgasmic—you almost certainly have the ability to have an orgasm, you just haven't had one *yet*. You're not allowed to declare, "I'm just one of those sad cases who can't have an orgasm," because chances are you just haven't found what works for you . . . yet! First, read and try everything this book suggests. Then, see whether a sex therapist can help. If after all that, you're still experiencing no orgasms, well, then maybe you are one of the rare unlucky ones. (There's information about possible medical causes of the problem on page 82.) But until you've tried it all, banish the thought!

If you're the partner of a preorgasmic person, trying to figure out how you can help, see page 83.

If you're single, there's zero reason to wait until you find a skilled partner to help you have your first orgasm. Start learning now—and then when that soulmate comes your way, you'll be ready for some incredible boomchickawowow together!

Why do most people with a clitoris find it easier to master having an orgasm themselves first, and then add orgasms to their partnered sex life? Well, if you're alone:

○ You have total control over the stimulation, so you can make the tiniest adjustments to hit your most sensitive spots exactly right (a half-millimeter to the left, a smidge more pressure, etc.) without even thinking about it, and definitely without having to ask for it.

○ You don't have to wonder what your partner thinks if it's taking a long time or worry if they yawn.

○ You'll be less likely to worry that your partner thinks you're a failure, or is losing interest in Project O, if there's no orgasm the first, third, or twenty-seventh time you try.

○ You don't have to fret about what your partner thinks of your backside, how recently you shaved your legs, or other thoughts that steal attention away from *enjoying* your body. (Hint: It is not easy to have an orgasm while sucking in your stomach.)

○ You won't be holding back out of concern about what you'll look like, what sounds you'll make, or what your partner will think when you're having an orgasm.

○ There's no chance that a partner's touch or words will be distracting at the wrong moment (this is possible even with the most caring, loving partner) since having an orgasm can sometimes require intense physical and mental concentration.

○ You won't be able to fool yourself by faking an orgasm.

When you're with a partner after you've had some orgasms on your own, you'll feel more confident and comfortable knowing exactly how it feels when you're very close to coming, and how it feels to allow yourself to "fall over the edge" into an orgasm. As you practice, you'll gain insights about what your body does and doesn't respond to, which could be handy to share with a partner later.

Okay, so you're alone. Choose times to work on this project when you won't be interrupted. Lock the door and put your phone on Do Not Disturb. Make yourself as comfortable as you can—you might want to put on sexy music, or start by taking a bath to relax.

Step Two: Befriend Your Vulva

Your v-friend is with you every minute of every day—it's time you got to know each other.

Your vulva is your external genitalia, the parts you can see without looking inside your vagina. It helps to have a clearer sense of what's there before you start asking these parts to help you have an orgasm. Take out a mirror or put your phone in selfie mode, sit back so you're resting on some pillows, set a light so you can see well, and take a look down there. You can prop up the mirror or phone on a pillow, or hold it with your feet.

A lot of us got the idea that penises are beautiful, even something to be worshipped (what's with all the phallic monuments?), but that vulvas are ugly, gross, disgusting, and smelly. Give us a break! Be prepared to discover something beautiful between your legs. A lot of people taking their first look are surprised to find that with the lips held apart, their vulva looks like a flower, a butterfly, a seashell, a heart, or an angel with spread wings. Vulvas are incredibly diverse: some larger or smaller, symmetrical or not, in all different shapes and intricately shaded browns, purples, and pinks. Would you recognize the face of your own vulva if you saw a photo?

Your outer lips, also called labia majora (the ones with hair on them—or where the hair used to be if you removed it) are easy to find. Locate your inner lips, too, called the labia minora. It's very common for some part of one or both inner lips to protrude outside the outer lips—either way (inner lips that stay hidden or friendly types that like to hang out) is totally normal. Do you have a neatly identical pair or a jaunty unmatched set? Both of those are normal too. Your inner lips are part of the larger structure of your clitoris and can be quite sensitive and feel lovely to touch.

My right labia minora is larger than my left one and I really thought this was ugly and unusual. It wasn't until college that I really started realizing my vulva was completely normal and beautiful.

I have a large vagina with meaty outer lips and I used to be self-conscious about it. But once my ex went down on me the first time, he loved it so much I had no shame in my game anymore!

Growing up with Barbie's genitals being a flat, labia-less crotch, it's easy to see why most girls are paranoid about their vulvas.

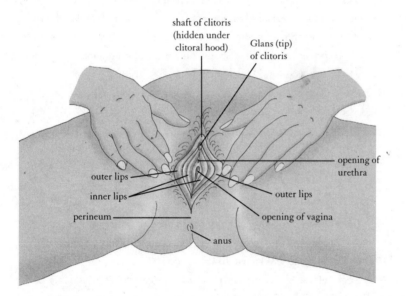

shaft of clitoris
(hidden under
clitoral hood)

Glans (tip)
of clitoris

opening of
urethra

outer lips

inner lips

outer lips

perineum

opening of vagina

anus

Up at the top, sort of where your outer and inner lips come together, find the glans (or head) of your clitoris. The part you'll see is like a bump—most are less than an inch long. You may need to pull back the hood of skin to make it visible. See whether you can feel the shaft of the clitoris (like the shaft of a penis) above the head—it feels like a small cord underneath the skin. Your clitoris continues inside your body—the entire organ is about the same size as a penis and has sensitivity throughout, but these external parts (glans and skin-covered shaft) are usually the most sensitive.

Porn Alert

PORN IS MESSING with people's concepts of what genitals are supposed to look like. Remember: The people hired to act in mainstream porn and those whose photos are online are cast because they have a specific body type—and genital type—that producers and website owners think people want to see. The same way that professionally produced mainstream porn nearly always features big penises and huge, often surgically enhanced breasts, vulvas in porn nearly always have the same basic "look." The look includes having inner lips that are pink, symmetrical, and smaller than the outer lips, and shaved pubic hair. If wannabe performers' genitals don't have the "preferred" size and shape, they either don't get the job, or they may get cosmetic surgery to change them.

Many people whose vulva *doesn't* look like the ones in porn worry that their body is abnormal or deformed.

Porn nearly always features symmetrical "tucked-in" labia minora, and for a long time as a young woman, I was unhappy with the way my vulva looked and it made me shy when sexually active.

There's even a growing industry of cosmetic surgery designed to make vulvas look more like the ones in porn, often by cutting off parts of the inner lips, a procedure known as labiaplasty.

Don't fall for it! Remember, porn may be entertaining for some people, but it's rarely an accurate source of information about sex, bodies, or what's "normal." Your inner lips are part of your clitoris—for some they're even more sensitive than the head of the clit. Surgically altering their shape won't help you have an orgasm. It may actually work against you, due to possible scar tissue and nerve damage caused by the surgery.

Rather than compare yourself to porn, check out the links and books listed on this book's website to get a much more accurate sense of what real bodies look like.

When I was younger, I noticed that my genitals didn't look like the ones in porn, and I was worried what my partners would think. As I got older, I realized mine are normal and it just didn't matter.

Growing up, I feared that my vulva and clitoris were too big and quite deformed. I used to watch porn to see if I was the only person who looked this way and I finally found a porn star who had a similar looking vag. It wasn't until my junior year that I finally did real exploration and learned that my genitals are perfectly normal. I also learned that porn stars' bodies are not the norm. It definitely made me more accepting and freer with my body. It helped me to enjoy vaginal and oral sex too.

Find your vaginal opening, the start of that incredibly elastic, muscular organ. A vagina can squeeze tightly around a finger or, with the right rush of hormones, expand its accordion-like folds to allow a baby to be born (and afterward, with the help of Kegel exercises, become toned enough to contract tightly again). To see exactly where your vagina is, you may want to wet your finger (licking it is the easiest way) and slide it inside an inch or so.

Just above your vagina, see whether you can see your urethral opening, the small hole where pee comes out. The skin just below your vagina is called the perineum. The hole below that is your anus.

I used to think all girl parts down there were gross, but since . . . really talking openly with friends in college, I love the vagina. It's awesome—weird looking, I guess, but in a fantastic way.

I was self-conscious for a while. I realized that the more I worried, the less enjoyment I was having and I wouldn't come. Every vagina is different and that is fine.

Step Three: Touch Yourself Experimentally. No Goal!

Step three isn't about having an orgasm. It's a way to do an easy little science experiment on your own body. Your goal is to find out what kinds of touch feel best to you, and what places on your body are most sensitive. You're especially interested in what kind of genital touching feels good.

Again, you want to be relaxed, so silence your phone and put on some nice music, take a bath or shower if you want. Start by running your hands all over your body in a way that feels good. Notice what areas feel nice to you. Caress your breasts and your nipples. Pay attention to the sensations.

After you've done this for a while, move your hand to your vulva (the external parts of your genitals, not inside your vagina). Touch around the different parts, noticing whether there are any areas that feel particularly nice when you touch them. Many people find their inner lips and urethral opening can be very pleasurable to touch. Because the clitoris is the part most likely to lead to orgasms, give it some particular attention. If you're not sure where it is, look back at page 61. See how creative you can be: How many different ways can you find to touch your clit? With each one, just notice: Does this feel more sensitive, or less? Does it feel good? Which side feels better? Would it feel better with a slightly lighter touch or slightly firmer? Try touching:

○ Directly on the head (the tip) of your clitoris
○ On the shaft rather than the tip
○ On the left side

- On the right side
- Side to side
- Up and down
- In circles
- Rolling the shaft of your clitoris under your finger
- With one finger
- With two fingers
- With tapping, massaging, stroking, and gentle pinching motions
- Any way you can think of!

Wet your fingers by putting them in your mouth, or adding some water-based lubricant, and then try touching some more. Most clits prefer wet fingers. Does yours?

If a partner has brought you to orgasm using their fingers but you've never been able to do it yourself, definitely experiment with touching yourself the way your partner does (or did). You can even imagine that it's your partner touching you as you use your own fingers.

If you want to, try putting a finger inside your vagina and experimenting with different ways of doing that. Do you like the sensation of having something inside you, or not so much? How does it feel if your finger moves? How about if you massage with your finger in different directions: up, down, left, right, at each different angle. Your anus also has lots of nerve endings—you can experiment with touching it, too, if you want. More on anal pleasure in Chapter 11.

Trying different speeds and pressure with my hand and moving around a lot helped me learn to have an orgasm. If one spot's not working, skip it and move on. Kind of like the SATs.

I would say exploration and experimentation are the best things to do when learning how to have an orgasm. Try everything you hear or read about. If you explore, you're bound to find something that satisfies you.

With each thing you do, just notice the sensations without judging yourself. If anything hurts or feels uncomfortable, stop doing that and try something else instead. You may feel very little at first, but pay attention to even the smallest sensations—they'll grow with practice. Try not to let any preconceived notions about what you *should* be feeling, or what you wish you were feeling, get in the way. Allow yourself to feel what you feel, and do more of the things that feel good.

I've found that turning my brain off and focusing on the pleasurable physical sensations makes a REALLY big difference. Sometimes this is easier to do than others. Being relaxed is also helpful.

Step Four: Keep Touching a Few Times Each Week. Experience Whatever Happens. Don't Give Up!

Now that you've spent some time observing what kind of touch your body likes best, keep doing it! Try to have a self-pleasuring/self-exploration session at least a few times a week—every day is fine if you like—for twenty minutes to an hour each time. (You probably happily shop, check your social media, or watch Netflix for that long a few times a week, if not daily; it's a perfectly reasonable amount of time to spend on something you enjoy.) Don't worry about trying to have an orgasm—just keep touching in the ways that feel good to you. You might find

Finding Your O After Gender-Affirming Surgery

FOR TRANS AND nonbinary people who've had gender-affirming surgeries, there can be a learning curve as you learn how your body has changed and what feels good. Depending on the type of surgery, the results will vary, but a lot of these same exploratory approaches can be useful in relearning your body. Obviously, also follow any post-op care recommended by your doctors! We'll discuss orgasm after gender-affirming surgery more in Chapter 9.

that you want to touch harder or faster as you get more turned on—if so, do it! Don't stress or worry about trying to make yourself have an orgasm, and don't let yourself start analyzing or judging yourself. If an orgasm comes along, great, but if not, just enjoy the pleasurable sensations.

It's a good idea sometimes to touch yourself with full awareness, paying close attention to the process. It can also help to touch yourself almost absentmindedly (when it's appropriate—we're not recommending you start doing it in the super-market canned goods aisle!). You could touch your clit or your whole body while you're alone watching TV, scrolling Instagram, or reading (whether or not what you're reading or watching is sexy). Let it be something you do sometimes for no reason at all, just because it feels nice.

Definitely don't stop doing these exercises, even if you've tried a few times and haven't had an orgasm. It can take a while for your body to "wake up" and start appreciating the sensations, and it can take a while for you to hone your technique. You may notice yourself getting aroused more on some days, less on other days. That's fine. When you do get aroused, keep doing the things that got you to that place. You're on the right track: orgasms happen at the peak of arousal.

Don't make having an orgasm a goal like trying to meet a productivity goal at work, where you work harder and harder and have less and less fun. Don't focus on orgasms while you're doing these exercises—instead, think about whatever you find hot, and whatever feels good. Enjoy the journey!

Step Five: Experiment with Other Things That Can Help Boost Your Arousal

- ○ **Squeeze the muscles of your vagina.** These are the same muscles you use to do Kegel exercises (see pages 34–36, 38). Squeezing and relaxing them speeds up your arousal and can help nudge you toward an orgasm. It's another thing to experiment with while you touch yourself.

Been There, Tried That, Didn't Like It

OKAY, SO YOU tried masturbating before and decided you didn't like it. Don't give up! The book *Tickle Your Fancy* wisely points out, "When you had sex for the first time, was it completely enjoyable? The first time you ate spinach...did you really like the taste?" Masturbation can be an acquired taste, and you'll get better as you practice. Don't write it off too fast.

○ **Move your hips.** Let them gyrate or thrust if it feels good. Move them up and back as you breathe and enjoy. Let your body move however it wants to.
○ **Relax and breathe.** You'll be able to feel more if you relax the muscles in your pelvis and genitals. Imagine breathing directly into your pelvis.
○ **Make noise.** Let yourself sigh, moan, and make whatever noises you feel moved to make.

For a long time I was worried I would be loud and someone would hear me, and that held me back from having an orgasm. Being confident no one can hear me helped.

○ **Use fantasy.** In our survey, 70 percent of orgasmic people with a vulva said they fantasized all or most of the time while they masturbated. By comparison, only 52 percent of vulva-owners who masturbated but hadn't yet had an orgasm said they always or often fantasized. Learning how to fantasize, or giving themselves permission to do so, is one of the most common things clitoris-owners say helped them learn to have an orgasm.

Use your imagination to find those images and stories that are sexy to you. Let your mind drift over them. You can replay the same moment over and over if it turns you on, or follow a whole story in your mind, making yourself one of the people in the story. You can pretend that your own hands are someone else touching you. Your fantasies are private thoughts—no one else can ever know what they are unless you tell them.

Don't stress about whether your conscious, analytic mind "approves" of the stories, and don't worry about whether you'd ever want to really do these things in real life. For now, they're just thoughts that turn you on—nothing more, nothing less. Most people of all genders use fantasy at least some of the time when they want to have an orgasm, especially when they're alone, and often when they're with a partner as well. For more about fantasy, and figuring out what fantasies you like, see page 38.

Creating my own "porn" in my mind helps me.

I watch porn almost always to get me in the mood and then I masturbate using my own fantasies/imagination.

○ **If you like, use erotica or porn.** If erotic stories (print or audio), romance novels, or porn arouse you, or the idea appeals to you, by all means, read or look at them while you touch yourself. If the idea turns you off, then don't! Some people have a strong preference for written or audio stories without images. Some like video but find it helps them to avoid mainstream fare and instead seek out independent porn, feminist porn, gay male porn, and other alternatives.

I enjoy listening to erotic audio! I think more people should be aware that sexy audio porn exists and it's GREAT. It feels way more intimate. That plus an active imagination equals wow.

When I discovered feminist porn, that changed everything for me.

I like using a vibrator and reading erotic fiction.

I prefer drawn porn over "real" porn (and drawn is preferably in comic form) and the story should be cute and all the characters are happy throughout.

Reading romance novels or something sexually stimulating is helpful prior to first touching myself. It helps me become aroused before masturbating.

○ **Try using a vibrator.** Vibrators create a different, more intense kind of sensation than your own fingers. Although not all clit-owners like how they feel, many find using one is by far the easiest way for them to have an orgasm.

My first vibrator was a liberating experience. I had masturbated for most of my life and had had several male sexual partners, but I never reached orgasm. My vibrator helped me take masturbation "over the top" and allowed me to finally fully release. In time, I learned to orgasm other ways and with a partner.

I prefer to be on my own with a vibrator so that I don't have to touch myself. I usually watch porn so that I don't have to pay too much attention to myself either.

I have an air pulse clitoral stimulator and it makes orgasms insanely quick and easy. I'd sincerely recommend it to anyone struggling to have an orgasm, and it's quite affordable!

If the idea appeals to you, get yourself a vibrator! In Chapter 7, read more about where to get one and how to use it.

○ **Keep your clit wet.** A woman recently came up to Dorian *before* one of our educational programs. She was beaming. "I'm so excited to be here!" she said. "I just had my first orgasm this week, and I'd been trying to have one forever!" After congratulating her, Dorian asked what she had done that had made the difference. "I used lube," the woman said. "You've got to tell people how much of a difference it makes to get things really good and wet." So, there you have it! Wet your fingers with saliva or lube at first. As you become aroused, if your vagina lubricates, you may be able to dip your fingers down and bring your own wetness up to your clitoris.

In order to have an orgasm, I had to learn to stimulate my other erogenous zones to get wet before trying to stimulate my clitoris.

Get Wet 'N' Wild

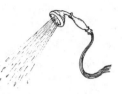

JETS OF WATER can be a great way to discover your orgasmic potential. If you have a handheld showerhead, try pointing it at your clit. You can also play with the jets in a Jacuzzi or the tub faucet (finding a position that works is the challenge there). We've heard from scores of people with a clitoris who owe their first orgasm (and their 101st) to a well-aimed stream of water, and at least two dozen of our vulva-owning survey respondents said it's their favorite way to come to this day.

I was taking a shower one day and pointed the water jet toward my vagina to rinse off soap. Luckily for me, it hit my clitoris and I discovered that I could achieve an orgasm that way. Each time I took a shower, I placed the jet on my clitoris until I couldn't stand it anymore; I wanted to take it off because the feelings were so overwhelming and unfamiliar, but it felt so good.

Running water on the clit is awesome! I like to do it lying down in the bathtub. There are no tools and you don't have to touch yourself if you're uncomfortable with that.

Things That Can Work Against You

If you're finding it hard to have an orgasm, check out this assortment of things that can work against you or slow you down. Do they ring true for you?

○ **Fear.** We always ask orgasmic audience members for their tips for others in the room who want to have an orgasm but haven't yet. "Don't be afraid!" is one of the most common answers. It's not unusual to feel apprehensive about the unknowns of orgasm, the intensity of the sensation, the sounds you'll make, what you'll look like, whether you'll feel embarrassed in front of your partner, or the possibility that you won't be able to have one. If you have a history of sexual trauma, the sensations of touch on your genitals, or of becoming aroused, could bring up powerfully negative memories or emotions. A sex therapist or the book *Healing Sex* by Staci Haines can be enormously helpful in working through these triggers.

Indeed, orgasms do involve a short loss of control and the vulnerability that comes with that. Most orgasmic people agree that an orgasm's deliciousness easily makes up for the things they used to worry about. Be bold and tap into that fearless part of yourself until your confidence comes more easily.

○ **Negative body image.** Some people walk around all day saying to their own body, "I hate you! You're fat, you're ugly, I hate everything about you!" and then turn around and say, "Okay, body, give me an orgasm." If this is you, don't be surprised when your body's reply is "Um, I don't think so. You hate me!" If your body hatred is intense, it can be difficult or impossible to allow yourself to experience physical pleasure—self-consciousness, insecurity, and dissatisfaction can shut down and prevent pleasure and orgasms. In an online Queendom.com survey of fifteen thousand people, 46 percent of women said self-consciousness about their body or hair was often what prevented them from having orgasms. A research study found that people of all genders who were anxious about their body tended to have lower sexual desire and enjoy sex less.

I am fat. I feel like there can be a lot of assumptions about fat bodies, and what fat folks genuinely like. There's a lot more to consider when having sex with fat bodies, such as positions, endurance, and assessing what feels good. For me, there has been a lot of unlearning of shame and embarrassment about what does and doesn't feel good.

Keep in mind that there are plenty of people whose body perfectly fits the cultural ideals, but whose self-consciousness prevents them from experiencing sexual pleasure. Many others have sex lives that are passionate and pleasure filled despite having a body shape that our culture denigrates. One's weight, appearance, or body type itself is actually irrelevant when it comes to sexual pleasure. What matters is how you think and feel about your body.

Body image is also an issue facing some—though certainly not all—people with physical disabilities. The cultural assumptions that disabled people don't, can't, or shouldn't have sex compound the problem. Some people living with disabilities face additional challenges, from limitations on what they're physically able to do, to the need for assistance or privacy from a care attendant, to pain or fatigue that can make sex difficult.

I've recently had to figure out how to have sex with a body that won't always do what it once did. I have to ask more for accommodations, which makes me feel less in control of things. I also just have waaaaay less energy and strength for everything.

The physical changes that come with childbirth, aging, and weight gain or loss affect body image for some people too. It can be tough to watch one's body change, especially if you feel that it's ever further from the cultural ideal—as unrealistic, youth obsessed, and unhealthy as that ideal may be. There's value in reminding oneself that these kinds of bodily changes—wrinkles, stretch marks, tummies that aren't flat, parts that sag—are normal, part of your story, and badges one earns for *being alive.* Who declared that only one narrow range of ages and skin tones and one narrow set of body types are beautiful? Who decided that ads and media would display endless young skin and figures, yet hide from us postpregnancy and elders' bodies, leaving so many feeling like their physical changes are some personal failure instead of part of the beauty of life? How dare those body-negative forces steal people's rights to experience pleasure in their body, just as it is?

Whatever your relationship with your body, befriending sometimes seems easier said than done. It's possible, however, to take steps toward negotiating a peace treaty. This may involve working with a therapist,

Dysphoria as a Barrier to Pleasure

EIGHTY-ONE PERCENT OF our trans and nonbinary survey participants said that at least sometimes, dysphoria gets in the way of their pleasure with or without a partner. Gender dysphoria can be described as any discomfort or distress one feels in relation to their gender identity not matching the sex assigned at birth. It does not necessarily mean a person "hates their body," and these feelings are not always constant but can be heightened in certain contexts. If a person isn't feeling comfortable with parts of their body, it's understandable that having those parts touched and stimulated might not be comfortable or welcome.

I don't want other people to derive pleasure from my body when I can't.

Although not all trans and nonbinary people experience dysphoria, it's a common barrier to pleasure since it can interrupt a person's relationship with their body. So, for trans and nonbinary people who experience dysphoria around their genitals, their chest, and other erogenous zones, it can be tricky to navigate pleasure. See page 231 for a few ideas on navigating this.

joining a body image support group, journaling, following body-positive or body-neutral social media accounts, or immersing yourself in great books about body image (see our suggestions at iloveorgasmsbook.com). Identifying role models whose body differs from the idealized thin, young, white, cisgender, able-bodied form but who still embody confident sexiness can be transformational.

Remind yourself that how you *feel* about your body matters far more in terms of your sexual pleasure than your body's actual size or shape.

One of the cool things about sex is that, for the most part, it works fine regardless of how you look. Having thinner thighs doesn't make you a better kisser. People with zits or gray hair can orgasm just as well as anybody else. Skin remains sensitive no matter what it looks like. Growing older usually brings with it more self-knowledge.

This is one of the themes of the emerging body neutrality movement, which encourages people to shift their focus away from how their body *looks* to focus on what it *does*. They say, instead of worrying that you're too critical of your body and feeling that you have to love it, take a neutral view toward it.

In some ways, sex (especially sex with yourself) is a chance to do just that: focus on the pleasure your body can give you, regardless of what it looks like.

> *Find partners who are positive about your body and make you feel gender euphoria with how they see you and compliment you and interact with you. Learn to love the parts of your body that you can, and try to enjoy those whenever possible.*

> *It made me sad that some day my body would get old and die, and I wouldn't experience it anymore. When I realized that sadness, I realized I didn't hate my body as much as I thought. I'm still dysphoric, but that doesn't mean I can't appreciate myself.*

○ **The belief that someone else should give you an orgasm.** If you have a vagina, chances are your orgasms are better and easier to come by if you're willing to take charge of your own climax. Don't assume an orgasm should be a gift one partner gives to another; most people with a

Speed Comes with Practice

YOUR FIRST ORGASM may take a long time to work up to, but rest easy. Most vulva-owners find they climax faster and more easily the more they practice. Not that the fastest orgasm is always the best, of course. But sometimes it is nice to be able to come before your fingertips are wrinkled prunes and you've developed a repetitive stress injury.

clitoris need to play an active role in seducing their own orgasm, sometimes with a partner who helps, sometimes not.

It took me a while to learn that penetration alone wouldn't induce an orgasm. Also, I couldn't expect the guy to know what he was doing—if I wanted to have an orgasm, I had to know how to position myself so I would have one. I have to take control.

○ **Concern about unplanned pregnancy, HIV, and sexually transmitted infections.** These are about the unsexiest things anyone could think about! Of course, these aren't risks during masturbation, but these issues can easily squelch an orgasm during partnered sex. When someone else's bodily fluids are involved, there's no such thing as sex with no risk at all (heck, there are risks to crossing the street, driving your car, and eating the leftovers in your fridge). But you *can* reduce the risks of sex—and allow yourself to relax and enjoy—with well-informed decisions about contraception and safer sex.

○ **Smoking, drinking, and medical conditions that affect circulation.** Sexual arousal and orgasm rely on blood circulation to the genitals. You might say, "If the blood don't flow, there ain't no O." Conditions like high cholesterol, high blood pressure, and coronary heart disease can have a negative impact on blood circulation, as can smoking, because it can cause blood vessels to constrict.

Drinking heavily has a numbing effect on nerve endings throughout your body, including down below. (Remember in old movies how they used whiskey for amputations before the invention of modern anesthesia?) Although some people find that a drink reduces sexual inhibitions, going overboard reduces your ability to feel sexual sensations. Numerous studies have discovered that with each additional alcoholic drink a woman drinks, the longer it takes her to have an orgasm, and the less intense the orgasm is. Penises are so prone to alcohol-induced challenges that the situation has its own slang: "whiskey dick." Our advice? Get so freaking comfortable with your sexuality that your sober self can be as wild and crazy as you like.

○ **Some medications.** One in six cis women in the US now take antide-pressants, along with one in eleven cis men and one in four transgender people. These drugs' potential for orgasm-inhibiting side effects pose a ballooning problem. Some people say the pharmaceuticals have no neg-ative side effects for them, but others find they reduce their sex drive, make it more difficult or impossible to come, or make their orgasms less intense or less satisfying. These issues create tough decisions for people taking the medications: It can be a painful conundrum to be forced to choose between having orgasms but being severely depressed or feeling good about life but never having an orgasm. Several people have told us they'd been suicidal before they found the right medication—they described their stark choice as nonorgasmic living versus death.

> *Being on antidepressants makes it extremely difficult for me to orgasm. It takes upwards of an hour and I can only seem to reach orgasm every couple of masturbation sessions.*

Hormonal methods of birth control (e.g., the pill, the patch, the ring, and Depo-Provera) can also have a negative impact on arousal and orgasm for some users although this varies depending on the person and the method.

> *I am grateful for [my birth control pills] every day and have no major side effects aside from the toll it has taken on my sex drive! It certainly is not anywhere near what it was before the pills.*

If your antidepressants, contraception, or other medications (anti-hypertensive, anticonvulsant, and antiulcer medication, as well as seda-tives, neuroleptics, and antihistamines, can all have similar side effects) are affecting your orgasms and you're frustrated by this, tell the doc-tor who prescribed them. Ask whether there are alternative options. Some antidepressant medications and some methods of hormonal birth control are less likely to have these side effects than others (although, unfortunately, some patients find that the antidepressants that work best for their depression are the ones with the negative sexual side effects).

For two years after she completed her primary cancer treatments, Dorian took a medication that reduced estrogen and testosterone production, based on evidence that this could reduce the risk of a cancer recurrence. We hope it did because it sure didn't spice up our sex life. During this period of time and in our conversations with others on other medications, we've learned two tips for trying to have orgasms on libido-crushing medications.

First, if you have orgasms sometimes but not as reliably as you'd like, see what you learn from the pattern of times you *have* been able to come. Was it twenty-three hours after you took the last pill, when the drug load was lowest in your body? (Some people on selective serotonin reuptake inhibitors, a.k.a. SSRIs, find it helps them to skip a dose, but this isn't safe for everyone—check with your provider before altering prescribed medication in any way.) Did it happen at a time when you were particularly aroused—maybe an especially long foreplay session, or some dirty talk that got you really hot? Was it a certain time during your menstrual cycle? (This may not apply if you're on hormonal contraception or hormone replacement therapy, a.k.a. HRT.) Finding and replicating the patterns won't make orgasms come easily, but it may help you maximize your chances of having one at all.

The second approach involves identifying tiny increases in your sexual arousal on any given day. People's sexual thoughts and interests naturally fluctuate over the course of each day. Let's say you graphed your "normal" (nonmedicated) sexual interests in a twenty-four-hour period. Maybe you wake up vaguely turned on by a sexual dream, then forget all about sex for a couple of hours, catch the eye of a cute barista as you pick up your morning coffee and entertain a few brief seconds of sexy thoughts, go to work, have a long stretch of nothing sexy at all until some sexual thoughts start flooding into your brain for no reason in the late afternoon and you get quite horny. A couple of hours later, you go home and, that evening, you notice mild arousal as you watch a sex scene in the series you've been bingeing. At the end of the day, you haven't had any sex or orgasms at all, but you could draw the lines on a graph, with small peaks (the coffee counter flirtation), high moments (that afternoon horniness with no explanation), and valleys (long morning at work).

On medication, your graph might look flatter, with fewer peaks, and the peaks of sexual interest you do have may be less intense. Still, you *will* have some mild peaks. Over the period of a few days or a week, notice when you have tiny upticks in sexual interest—start a note on your phone and jot it down if that would help you remember. Then, start looking for patterns. Do you tend to have your most sexual thoughts in the mornings or at night? In the middle of your menstrual cycle, or just before or after your period? Is there some visual trigger during the day that creates the littlest spark? Rather than feeling sorry for the ravenous urges you know you're *not* feeling, find ways to catch your little peaks and ride them for all they're worth. Vibrators can also be particularly useful for clit-owners with decreased sensitivity.

While these approaches help some people some of the time, others choose to make peace with their lack of orgasms. Cuddling, sensual touch, massage, and other kinds of physical intimacy can be extremely pleasurable without an orgasm, and these shift the focus from what you're *not* feeling to the joy of the sensation you do feel.

Additional Advice from Trans and Nonbinary People

FOR TRANSGENDER AND nonbinary people, orgasms might flow easily—or they might not. In our survey, 90 percent of trans and nonbinary people had had orgasms through masturbation, and 57 percent had during partnered sex. We asked for their advice to other trans and nonbinary people who may be learning to have an orgasm, and received so much wisdom. These seven distinct themes emerged.

1. **Explore your body with curiosity and patience.** Give yourself the gift of patience and plenty of time. "Take your time" was the most frequently offered piece of advice! There's no deadline and there need not be a goal.

It took me a long time to figure it out on my own! I thought I was broken, but it just took patience and learning about my body.

Don't let the world into your most intimate pleasures. Take a deep breath and explore slowly, lovingly.

2. **Let go of your preexisting assumptions about what masturbation "should" look like.** Pleasuring your body doesn't have to be genital focused. Bodies have infinite erogenous zones, so explore everywhere. Experiment with ways to touch your body and your genitals. Discover what feels good.

    Most of what we consume is so focused on genitals that it neglects knowing all the skin you're in, what brings joy and what definitely doesn't.

    Touch yourself the way that makes sense to you. You might not get anything from touching yourself the way other people of your gender do, because your anatomy might be different. And you might not like touching yourself the way other people with your anatomy do, because they are mostly a different gender than you. Figure out what works for your body and your brain.

3. **You may choose to use strategies specifically to avoid thinking about, looking at, and/or touching your own body.** If dysphoria stands in the way of sexual pleasure, these kinds of workarounds can be a breakthrough.

    If you need to not think about your body, then don't think about it. Go somewhere else in your head. Put a barrier between you and your genitals. You can always work up to being more engaged with your body, but don't feel like you have to start there.

    I would recommend turning the lights off, putting a blanket over yourself so that you don't have to see anything, and maybe finding sex toys or objects that you can use so that you don't have to touch yourself.

4. **Toys and accessories can help.** Using sex toys can be fun for anyone, but toys and gender gear can be especially helpful for trans and nonbinary

folks. A toy or accessory can be a way to pleasure your body without touching it, as well as a way to engage your imagination as you explore. (More about toys and gender gear in Chapter 7.)

5. **You don't need penetration.** A lot of trans masculine people may not enjoy or desire penetration. Since penetration is not an effective route to orgasm for the vast majority of people with a vagina, you're not missing out! Find what works and feels best for you.

6. **Remind yourself that you are deserving of pleasure.**

   Remember that loving yourself is so so important. If you don't love and explore your own self, it will be that much harder to accept love and know how to communicate your sexual needs/wants to others.

   Humans were given the gift of feeling sexual pleasure, and this gift is taken away from us by biological essentialists telling us all sorts of terrible things about our identities and making us feel guilty for not feeling comfortable in the labels they forced upon us. Having an orgasm by yourself is a political act. It's a way of refusing gender dysphoria—refusing the pain that we feel due to what exterior forces expect of us—and accepting our inner and outer beauty.

7. **Enjoy the journey; let go of the goal.** Embrace pleasure for pleasure's sake. Whether an orgasm happens need not be a goal.

   No pressure! Coming isn't always the point of masturbating so let it be a nice bonus rather than the only reason you're doing it.

Orgasms with a Partner

ONCE YOU'VE HAD some orgasms on your own, if you're in a relationship or craving a hookup, you may be raring to have them with a partner. Your knowledge that your body is fully capable of coming should give you a confidence boost, but that doesn't mean it's always easy to have an orgasm with a partner. It may take a

Could It Be a Medical Problem?

IF YOU'VE TRIED the types of techniques discussed in this chapter and you're still not having orgasms, it's possible there's a medical explanation. Vulva-owners can ask their doctors for a pituitary function test (prolactin level) and a fasting blood sugar. These two blood tests can reveal medical issues that can impair your ability to have an orgasm, according to sex therapist Judith Seifer, PhD, professor of sexual health at the Institute for Advanced Study of Human Sexuality.

For people with a vulva who used to have orgasms but can't anymore, Dr. Seifer finds that common physical causes include multiple sclerosis, lupus, Addison's disease, adult-onset diabetes with neuropathy, and some collagen diseases. If you're living with one of these diagnoses, a doctor or a sex therapist (see page 86) may be able to help you explore your options.

If you have a penis and orgasms or erections have become harder (pun intended) to come by, Chapter 10 has troubleshooting advice.

while to learn how to come now that you're adding on the elements of:

○ Having someone looking at you
○ Having your body touched or stimulated in ways you're not controlling
○ Having more going on in your head: Should I be pleasuring my partner? What do they think? Am I taking too long? Is this going to work? Not to mention the random conversations that pop up when two people are together.

Just because your body has now had orgasms doesn't mean you'll come at the drop of a hat (or should we say the drop of some undies?). You'll probably need to make sure that at some point during the interaction you get some good, sustained clitoral action, whether that's from oral sex, your own hand, your partner's hand, a vibrator, or maybe rubbing against your partner's body. Don't worry about "being greedy"—sex is about both giving and receiving, not always simultaneously. You should have plenty of time to receive sexual pleasure! Most people with a vulva who have orgasms during partnered sex play find they need to be assertive and "take charge of their own orgasm" if they want to make sure it'll happen.

Especially while you're still learning, you may find it helps to ask your partner to cut back on "distracting" caresses to let you focus on the key sensations that may get you off. Having them kiss you, suck on your nipples, or thrust deep inside you may feel great, but for some people with a vulva, it sends them in a different direction, away from their climb toward climax. If you suspect this is the case, try saying something like "You feel so good....What you're doing with my clit is so hot, it might make me come—if I can just focus on that one sensation for a while, so I don't get distracted—yes, just like that!" There's more specifically about having orgasms during penis-in-vagina sex in Chapter 5.

Ideally you have a supportive, patient partner who knows that this is new for you, will help you get the stimulation you need, and won't make a big deal if it takes a bunch of attempts over a period of time to get the hang of things. Without that comfort and communication, it can be a lot more challenging, though not impossible, in a first-time hookup situation with someone you don't know well. With any partner you hope to be with again, this is not the time to start faking—then, you'll *really* confuse matters if you want to try for real the next time. Don't forget to enjoy being sexual whether or not you have an orgasm. Figuring out how to have orgasms together can be a fun joint project, but it doesn't have to be your main goal; don't let it eclipse the physical and emotional pleasure of being together.

Troubleshooting: Wimpy Orgasms

I have orgasms, but they're so little and pathetic. How can I have orgasms with "POW!"?

Kegel exercises (pages 34–36, 38) can be the key to bigger, better orgasms—with comic book "POW!" as one audience member once described them. For both penis- and vulva-owners, getting your PC muscles in shape can bolster their ability to contract more intensely during your orgasms, resulting in more sensation for you. Avoiding quickies, and instead spending more time with long buildups (as in the game on page 102), can also give you bigger blast-offs.

First Orgasm Tips for Partners

YOUR PARTNER'S NEVER had an orgasm? Here are some ways you can help:

○ Enjoy sex together without making orgasm your goal. Your partner is much more likely to have an orgasm in your presence if they're enjoying themselves. Being obsessively focused on making your partner come— rather than just helping them feel pleasure—can take the joy out of sex.

Partners' Attitudes Matter

MAYBE SAYS: FOR a lot of trans and nonbinary people, gender dysphoria can be activated or increased by how others perceive us. So, in sexual relationships, the way a partner interacts with our body can quickly shift how we respond to the interaction. It's very obvious to me when a partner is misgendering me with their touch or the way they're navigating my body. Without them saying a word, I can quickly tell whether they're affirming me in their thoughts or they're not. And that largely influences how comfortable I'm going to feel in that interaction.

Sometimes I get into phases of deep dislike for my body that gets in the way of me enjoying any physical activities. My distrust of how others treat me and my body has also prohibited me from seeking out partners in the past.

Being partnered with someone who understands, accepts, and celebrates my nonbinary identity led me to my first orgasm because I was able to finally focus on pleasure rather than my perception.

Know that their ability to have an orgasm with you likely has nothing to do with whether they love you or enjoy sex with you.

○ Spend lots of time on activities that focus on your partner's pleasure, particularly those that stimulate the clitoris. Oral sex can work well, but only if they're comfortable with it. See Chapter 4.

○ If your partner's never had an orgasm, encourage them to explore on their own, and then incorporate it into sex with you once they've figured it out. Some people don't masturbate because they're worried about what their partner would think, so make sure yours knows they have your support.

○ Give your partner this book, or the others we recommend on this book's website, to give them ideas of what to do.

○ If they want to have their first orgasm with you, or they've had orgasms through masturbation but never with a partner, be exceptionally patient. Having an orgasm with someone else in the room can be like the experience of being "pee-shy," where it's hard to urinate with another person present. Realize it will get easier and faster with practice. Don't add to the pressure they're probably putting on themselves to make it happen. Communicate things like "If it happens this time, great, and if not, that's fine, it'll happen some other time" and "We can take as long as you need and keep going as long as it feels good."

> *The first guy I had sex with couldn't please me; he wasn't patient. The guy I'm dating now has been a blessing. He's very patient, lets me try whatever positions I want, talks to me about what I like, then does it. I guess I had to learn to be comfortable with the person I'm with in order to have an orgasm.*

○ If they've had orgasms before but never with a partner, do what you can to replicate their masturbatory conditions until they get the hang of you being part of it. If they always come while lying on their back, have them lie on their back. If they use their fingers on their clit, have them do that. If they use a vibrator, they can use the vibrator during sex with you. Let them get accustomed to coming in their "original way" while you touch or pleasure them; later you can expand your repertoire together so they can come in a wider variety of ways.

○ If shyness, guilt and shame about sex, a history of abuse or assault, body image issues, or a sex-negative upbringing get in the way of your partner's ability to enjoy sexual pleasure, there are no overnight cures, but you can certainly help. With honesty and respect, compliment whatever aspects of your partner's body and genitals are attractive or sexy to you (don't lie—they'll be able to see right through that). Your partner may brush aside your comments or think you couldn't possibly mean what you're saying, but over time, they may start to accept the idea that you find them attractive (even down below), and rethink the way they think about themselves.

I felt uncomfortable about the appearance of my vagina up until a few years ago because one side of my labia is bigger than the other. It wasn't until I saw pictures of sexually mature women, read educational materials, and had a loving boyfriend who adored my vagina that I came to love it. I think I look like a beautiful, sexually mature woman.

○ Cultivate a mutually curious, exploratory attitude toward sex in your relationship. Never push your partner beyond their comfort zone, but do explore anything sexual that interests them (as long as it's safe and comfortable for you). Read books about sex together—choose ones they say appeal to them—and discuss what you read. Attend workshops and classes about sex to learn more together—make it a fun date. Our top picks for resources about healing from sexual abuse, and helping a partner heal, are on page 49.
○ Realize that ultimately, this needs to be your partner's own process of learning about their own body. While you can help and be supportive, you can't do it for them.

For More on Finding Your O

LOOKING FOR MORE in-depth instruction on how to find your O? There are entire books on the subject, or you might find it helpful to work with a sex therapist. You'll find links and titles at iloveorgasmsbook.com.

3

Petting the Bunny
Masturbation and Orgasm

Masturbation is the fastest and easiest way for many clitoris-owners to have orgasms, and the most common way for them to come for the first time. In our survey, those who had masturbated were far more likely to be orgasmic than those who had never masturbated (93 percent compared to 35 percent). And, of course, there's the old joke about penis-owners: 98 percent masturbate, and the other 2 percent are lying. (That's an exaggeration, but there's truth to the fact that every study of people with a penis finds very high rates of solo sex.) With no disease risk and no chance of accidentally knocking or getting knocked up, self-pleasuring clearly has a lot going for it.

This chapter's primary focus is on people with a clitoris, since they're the ones who receive the lion's share of anti-masturbation shame, stigma, and lack of information. One historic moment that illuminated how this so often played out is when former US surgeon general Joycelyn Elders recommended that American children should receive comprehensive age-appropriate sex education that included information about masturbation. Her statements came under fierce attack and ultimately led to her forced resignation. In news commentary, TV host David Brinkley asked why "twelve-year-old boys should be taught skills they already have." Columnist Richard Goldstein pointed out in response that if masturbation were discussed in school, *girls* would learn about it too. It was the potential to promote sexual pleasure for clitoris-owners that made the subject so threatening to so many people, and sadly, not enough has changed in the intervening years.

I knew some of my friends masturbated, but in general, I didn't have much of a sex drive and wasn't interested in sex with myself or others of any sort. It wasn't until I was twenty that I first masturbated (two years after I first had sex), and after that, I realized that I was FAR better at making myself happy than anyone else was!

In my older years, and as I've come to understand myself as nonbinary, masturbation has been an amazing way to heal my relationship with my body. It's purely sensation based—sometimes I focus on my body or my energy, sometimes I think about the sky or trees. It's an incredible release of physical and emotional tension. It's a holy time for me.

For people with a clitoris, masturbation can be culturally complicated. Some are practically masturbation cheerleaders; others enjoy self-loving privately but would be horrified to discuss the matter. Still others don't masturbate at all, for a variety of reasons.

I don't feel like touching myself sometimes, and sex or masturbation can give me bottom dysphoria.

I never took a negative stance toward masturbation because my mother encouraged exploration of one's body, as long as it was behind closed doors. However, I also never took advantage of masturbation; it was simply something I wasn't interested in.

Whatever anyone's individual situation, the taboo against masturbation for people with a vulva is powerful. Not only do kids assigned female at birth get the message that they're not supposed to do it, they're not even supposed to acknowledge that they *can* masturbate. Confusion is rampant. One woman told us that growing up she heard that masturbation was "touching yourself," so she assumed she was masturbating anytime she scratched her ear or touched her arm. Another said she got the idea that masturbation required a large, expensive machine. "I was just a little kid," she said, "so I couldn't afford one of those machines. But I figured maybe I'd get one when I grew up."

People start absorbing information about this subject from the time they're babies. Parents often move babies' hands away from their genitals and don't teach them the words for that part of the body—a very different reaction than when the same baby explores their belly, ears, or toes. If this happens repeatedly, the baby quickly comes to the conclusion that this part of their body is "bad" or that touching it is "wrong." As adults, most of us don't have conscious memories of infancy. Yet feelings of shame can run deep, sometimes because they were planted so early, and sometimes because we live in a culture saturated with negative messages.

These messages often persist through childhood. One person shared that when they were little, any time they or their siblings put their hands anywhere near their genitals, their mother would say, "That's dirty! Move your hand!" Another remembers that after a day at the beach when she was a girl, she was in the outdoor showers with her mom and sisters. When she reached down to dump out the sand that had collected in the crotch of her bathing suit, her mom slapped her hand away, saying, "Get your hand away from there!" The take-home message that many kids learn is simple: Your genitals are nasty. Don't touch them. If you take any interest in them at all, you're a bad person.

Some vulva-owning kids follow instructions, not getting to know much about their own body and sexuality—and often discover they have a *lot* of catching up to do as adults. Other kids look and touch in secret, sometimes overwhelmed with shame and guilt. Most adults with a vulva tell us that if the subject of masturbation came up in conversation when they were teens, they'd squeal, "Eeewww, disgusting!" and swear they didn't do it—whether or not it was true. As one nineteen-year-old wrote on our survey:

Any time my friends talk about masturbation it's followed by giggles and "Ewwwwww—God no!" Yet in the back of my mind I'm thinking, "I LIKE IT!" I'm scared to say that out loud because it's like masturbation is looked down upon.

To make matters worse, there's a massive double standard that says masturbation is something kids with a penis do, and kids with a vagina don't. Some kids heard that masturbation is bad for everyone—but that "boys can't control themselves," so people make an exception for them. As a kid, one woman heard that if boys didn't masturbate, they'd explode. (We can just imagine the seventh grader sitting in a classroom, watching the thirteen-year-old at the next desk self-combust in a fiery explosion. "Poor thing," she'd think to herself. "He really should have taken care of that.")

My father mentioned masturbation as though it was normal for boys but only "certain kinds of girls" did it.

I was told that it was for boys to do. I never did it; I wouldn't have known how to. Since I thought it was only for boys, I never really thought about trying to do it.

On average, people with a penis (kids and adults) do masturbate more than those with a vulva do, but rates of reported clitoris-and-vagina-based solo sex have been on the rise for decades. Penises happen to be *way* easier for their owners to discover, the way they just hang out down there, so easy to see and touch. Vulvas and vaginas, by comparison, are tucked away where they're less visible. It's a handy place to keep one's genitals, but it means that it often takes a while longer to discover one's clitoris. Penis-owners even have to touch their genitals every time they pee. If clitoris-owners had to touch their clit every time they peed, they'd be ten thousand times more familiar with that part of their body. This puts those with a clitoris at a huge disadvantage.

These days, growing numbers of parents are teaching their kids the real words for the sex organs, communicating that these parts are healthy and normal, and even letting their kids know that masturbation is perfectly okay (in private, not at the dinner table).

My mother explained to me what masturbation was when I brought it up. She told me that there was nothing wrong with it, that everyone does it at some point, and that I should enjoy the pleasure I can give myself.

What's a Parent to Do?

MANY PARENTS TELL us, "I don't want to raise my kids the way my parents raised me, but what am I supposed to do when one of them is on the playground rubbing themselves up and down against the swing-set pole? Or when we have dinner guests and my kid is walking around with both hands down their pants?"

The key for parents is to communicate to their kids that touching oneself is something that's okay to do, but only in private, like in their bedroom or the bathroom at home. Rather than yelling, "Get your hands out of there!" a parent can quietly say to a child, "I know it feels good to touch there, but that's something people do in private. You can do it in your room later if you want to." That way, parents teach their kids appropriate behavior without inadvertently sending the message that touching your own body is fundamentally wrong.

When I was in about sixth grade, I told my mom about touching myself. I felt extremely guilty about it and I almost started to cry, fearing that I was doing something horribly wrong. She laughed a little bit and then told me there was nothing wrong with what I was doing, that it was perfectly natural and most people do it.

My mom always told me that the only way somebody will ever really please you sexually is if you know your body well enough to know what you like. So she encouraged masturbation. She bought me my first vibrator when I was sixteen.

Clearly, though, too many still grow up steeped in masturbation stigma. Because the subject is so forbidden, millions of people with a clitoris, in particular, spend decades—or lifetimes—denied basic knowledge about their own body and the pleasure that comes with it. It's time to kiss this taboo good-bye!

What's the Fastest and Easiest Way for Vagina-Owners to Have Orgasms?

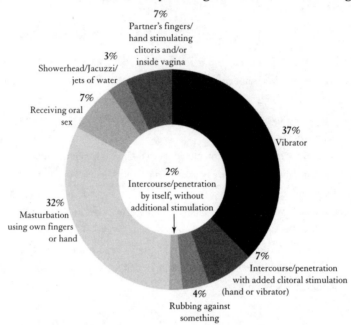

7%
Partner's fingers/
hand stimulating
clitoris and/or
inside vagina

3%
Showerhead/Jacuzzi/
jets of water

7%
Receiving oral
sex

37%
Vibrator

2%
Intercourse/penetration
by itself, without
additional stimulation

32%
Masturbation
using own fingers
or hand

7%
Intercourse/penetration
with added clitoral stimulation
(hand or vibrator)

4%
Rubbing against
something

Eight Lies You May Have Heard About Masturbation

YOU'LL PROBABLY RECOGNIZE most of these as the falsehoods they are. Maybe some of them still make you nervous, though. All eight come up regularly from our audience members, who say they're things they've heard and sometimes worried about. Let's put these long-lived fictions to rest once and for all!

Lie #1

If you masturbate, you won't be able to have an orgasm with a partner.

Truth: The reverse is true. Studies find that in general, people with a clitoris who've had orgasms through masturbation are much more likely to have orgasms during partnered sex, and that those are more likely to be frequent and multiple. There are lots of reasons: People who are comfortable touching their own body are more likely to know what feels good to them sexually. They're less likely to be surprised by or afraid of the sensations as they near orgasm. And they may be better able to let their partner know what they like. Not only does solo sex pose no danger to your partnered sex life, it just might improve it.

Recently, my husband and I were having some issues in the bedroom. My mother asked if I had ever orgasmed with my husband. Unfortunately, my answer was no. She basically told me that he wouldn't know how to pleasure me unless I knew what felt good. That way, I could take my educational experience and share it with him. It worked!

Lie #2

Masturbation will change the way your genitals look—and then everyone will know you've been doing it.

Truth: You can't change the shape of your clitoris or labia (inner or outer vaginal lips) by masturbating with your hand, a vibrator, or anything else (unless your technique involves sharp objects!). It's impossible for any doctor or partner to know, by examining you, whether you masturbate. The only exception would be if your skin temporarily got red or irritated from rubbing, but you could see and feel the tenderness if that happened.

For penis-owners, perhaps to the disappointment of some, you're not going to lengthen the shaft by pulling on it. If that were true, the streets would be full of those whose pride and joy hung below their knees. It's possible that a particular self-love technique, over the course of many years, might create or exacerbate a slight curve to the penis. But since curves are common and it's rare for any penis to be perfectly straight, a curved penis is not going to out you as a masturbator.

Where did all this worry come from? Many young adults take a close look at their clitoris, labia, penis, or some other part, notice something about it ("It's big!" "It's small! "It's lopsided!") and decide that this must be the result of touching themselves too much. It's an understandable assumption, but it's incorrect. You can read more on vulva diversity on pages 60–64.

Many people discover masturbation around the time that puberty hits. Most people with a vulva know that they'll develop breasts and get their periods; they may not realize that during puberty labia also often grow and change. If you've been masturbating, it can be easy to assume it's the masturbation that caused the labia to look different rather than the hormones racing around your body.

The shape, size, and asymmetry of your genitals have nothing to do with whether or how you touch them. In fact, like every other part of your body, they probably look a lot like your relatives' genitals. (Now *there's* a Thanksgiving conversation starter!)

Hymens: The Unbroken Truth

MOST OF WHAT you've heard about the hymen is a myth. Contrary to conventional wisdom, it's not an inch or two inside the vagina, lying in wait to be broken like a sheet of plastic wrap. According to Hanne Blank in her fascinating book *Virgin: The Untouched History*, the hymen is simply the skin that connects the inside of the vagina to the outside of the body. It's quite rare for it to entirely or mostly cover the opening of the vagina, so usually there's nothing at all to break or tear. In some cases there's a small amount of tissue there that could bleed a little, but more often if there's some bleeding it's the result of not using enough lube rather than damage to any hymen tissue. Unless you find it extremely uncomfortable or impossible to insert a finger or a tampon, you can probably pretend you never even heard of the hymen. Odds are, it won't have any impact on your experience of first-time penetration.

It's also impossible to tell whether someone has masturbated or had penetrative sex or not based on the appearance of the hymen. Right from the start, before anyone has any kind of sex, hymens look so different that the state of your hymen can't tell anything about you.

I ♥ ORGASMS

Lie #3

Masturbation is only for single people.

Truth: Yes, single people masturbate. So do people in relationships and people who are married. Lots of couples use their hands or fingers to stimulate each other's genitals, or take turns by having one partner masturbate themselves while the other "helps" by caressing, kissing, licking, stroking, telling sexy stories, or otherwise further arousing the one doing the masturbating. Some find masturbation is a great way for a horny partner to get off without imposing on a partner who's not in the mood. Even if they don't masturbate together, lots of partners do so when they're apart—can you say, "long distance relationship"? This might happen on their own, or together via video chat. One college student said that the only way she's ever been able to come is while her boyfriend talks dirty to her on the phone (and she touches herself at the same time).

Lie #4

(or at least, not as clear-cut as you might think)

The Bible says masturbation is a sin.

Truth: Bible experts are in disagreement on this one. Basically, there's one Bible story that people usually point to as evidence that the Bible says masturbation is wrong, the story of Onan in Genesis 38:7–10. In the story, Onan's brother dies. The law at the time (biblical times, remember) requires Onan to have sex with his dead brother's wife, so as to produce an heir for his brother. Onan refuses—instead, he "spills his seed on the ground." For this offense, God strikes Onan dead. Yes, Onan was punished for a big-time crime, but most modern Bible scholars say his crime wasn't masturbation but his unwillingness to procreate with the widow. (The story even suggests that this may have been a case of "pulling out," not masturbating.) Beyond that, many scholars say, the Bible says nothing specific about masturbation at all.

Writer and poet Dorothy Parker is said to have joked that her parakeet was named Onan because he spilled his seed on the ground.

There is similar disagreement about how to interpret Buddhist, Muslim, and other Christian and Jewish scriptures and teachings about masturbation. Overall, two things are clear: First, masturbation by anyone with a vulva is rarely, if ever, mentioned in the sacred texts of any of these faiths. Second, many respected leaders within these religious traditions say masturbation is perfectly acceptable within their faith, at least in some circumstances.

Lie #5

You can hurt yourself or damage your body by masturbating.

Truth: Obviously, anything can be risky if you don't use common sense. Case in point: Pleasuring yourself while driving is dangerous, no matter how much it might liven up a boring cross-country trip. We don't recommend it. What you do in the backseat is, of course, your own business.

Lie #6

A person who masturbates will no longer be a virgin.

Truth: The concept of virginity is built on ideas about purity and penetration. People may define it differently based on many different cultural factors, but most agree that notions of "losing" it mean participating in sexual activities with a partner. Masturbation is a solo activity, and plenty of virgins touch themselves. For some people who are choosing not to have intercourse, masturbation helps them satisfy their sexual urges. Nine in ten virgins who took our survey say they've masturbated.

Lie #7

Only lesbians/sluts/bad girls masturbate.

Truth: Let's set the record straight about what kinds of people with a vulva commonly masturbate:

- Heterosexuals. Bisexuals. Lesbians. Those who describe themselves as "none of the above." Cisgender people. Transgender people. Nonbinary people.
- People who have lots of sex. Those who've never had sex with a partner. Those who wish they were having more partnered sex than they are. Those who aren't interested in partnered sex.
- People who are single, married, and dating. Those who aren't sure if that person they hook up with sometimes is officially a "relationship" or not.
- People of every age, race, ethnicity, and religious denomination. Atheists and agnostics too.

Lie #8

You need to be careful not to masturbate too much.

Truth: If you're not showing up for work, standing up your friends, or avoiding your significant other because you're too busy self-pleasuring, then you're overdoing it. Otherwise, there's nothing to worry about! It's perfectly fine for a person to masturbate every day or several times a day. It's also fine to masturbate less or not at all. Most people find they go through phases depending on their mood, menstrual cycle, stress level, relationship status, and other factors—there's no right or wrong frequency when it comes to self-pleasure. After all, people don't worry about getting "addicted" to other enjoyable, perfectly healthy pastimes like rock climbing, doting on houseplants, or practicing the latest viral dance moves.

It may also be helpful to separate "masturbating too much" from "watching too much porn." For many people, these two activities go hand in hand (sorry, couldn't help ourselves), but they don't have to. If you're going to worry about doing something "too much," porn should be the one giving you pause. Watching mountains of porn risks filling your mind with unrealistic expectations for sex, reducing your interest in being with a real live partner, and possibly affecting your self-esteem and body image. On the other hand, just diddling daily (or several times a day) using fantasy as your inspiration is generally harmless.

Porn You Can Feel Good About?

FOR MANY PEOPLE (66 percent of our survey respondents), porn is part of their masturbation experience at least some of the time. Some are perfectly happy with the universe of mainstream porn: they understand it's entertainment, not real life, the offerings suit their taste, and it does the job of getting them off.

Plenty of others are frustrated with or critical of mainstream porn for a wide variety of reasons. Maybe they feel that:

- There's not enough of a plot to engage them.

- It's too violent or aggressive.

- It's overly focused on male pleasure.

- Its representation of what most women enjoy and how most women want to be treated sexually is laughable.

- The narrow slice of body and genital "types" featured make them feel badly about themselves.

- It encourages them to think about how they look instead of how they feel.

- It's full of racist, heteronormative, and cisnormative stereotypes.

- They don't feel good about the porn industry and how it treats its performers.

- Or maybe it just doesn't turn them on!

Experiences with the big, conventional porn sites send some people to search for options they can feel better about. The good news is that because of consumer demand, there are now lots of sites that market themselves differently. Some are designed by and for women, or by and for queer people. Some show real-life "amateur" couples having sex, instead of actors. Some are full-length films with high-quality cinematography. Some aim to be sensual rather than explicit. Some allow customers to pay performers directly to create the kind of porn they enjoy.

Free porn misleads. If you pay for porn, you can get shit aligned with what actually turns you on and can help you expand on what you like.

Ethically made porn is a lot more realistic, shows real intimacy, even giggling or playfulness that doesn't exist in mainstream porn.

I feel like consuming feminist porn has actually reversed some of the damage done by the mainstream porn I consumed in my youth. Seeing realistic bodies having actual sex that looks fun and empowering has helped me feel good about acting on my own fantasies and feeling good about my own body during sex.

How to Masturbate: The Missing Manual for People with Clits

TIME AND TIME again, clitoris-owners have told us, "I wanted to masturbate when I was growing up—I just didn't know how to do it." One said that when she was little, her mom gave her a kid's book about sexuality. The book said masturbation was healthy and normal, and the child thought to herself, "Oh, good, now I can finally learn how to do it!" She turned the page expecting to find step-by-step instructions—but the book had already moved on to a new subject.

In middle school and high school I masturbated by insertion and I never achieved orgasm. It wasn't until college that I discovered my clitoris and orgasm. I think this was all due to lack of information on the subject.

I wanted to masturbate but had no idea how to. It wasn't until after I got to college and had the privacy of my own computer to find websites geared toward women who also didn't know how. I was surprised to find that I wasn't frigid and that I was quite good at it.

Anywhere from 10 to 30 percent of the vulva-owners in our audiences say they didn't masturbate as kids because they had no idea how to do it. Between 80 and 90 percent say they were told *nothing* about masturbation when they were growing up. Some figure things out on their own, or with the help of a friend, big sister, or book. Others reach young adulthood before they learn how to do it.

How do vulva-owners do it? A *lot* of different ways! They might:

- Touch, rub, or stroke their clitoris, especially the shaft (see diagram on page 61), using one or two fingers. This is the most common way people who have a clitoris masturbate.
- Use a vibrator to stimulate their clitoris (more on this in Chapter 7)
- Touch, rub, stroke, or massage other parts of their genitals, like their labia, urethra, or anus
- Use water to stimulate their clit: a handheld showerhead or the jet of water from a Jacuzzi or bathtub faucet
- Squeeze their thighs together
- Insert a finger or fingers, sex toy, or another object in their vagina
- Caress, massage, or squeeze their breasts and/or nipples
- Build up muscular tension by tightening muscles all over their body
- Rub their clitoris against something, like a pillow, pile of blankets, or piece of furniture
- Fantasize by thinking about a story that turns them on, or imagining an image or memory that's sexy to them

Of course, people also mix and match, using different approaches in one self-lovin' session, or playing different ways on different days. And some choose not to have solo sex at all, which is okay too.

I still don't really masturbate—I've never gotten the hang of it. I do remember discovering that I could touch myself and that it felt good, but I've never been good at actually turning myself on or giving myself an orgasm.

"I've always had a dream of making a book called *There's No Right Way to Masturbate.*"
—actress and film producer Shailene Woodley

As an ace [asexual] person, I never crave sex, but I feel like I would be open to it if genitals didn't just weird me out. My gender dysphoria has really turned me away from self-pleasure.

Why is it so hard to find complete, illustrated, step-by-step "How to Masturbate" instructions for people with a vulva? Mostly because there are so many different ways. A technique that makes one person's toes curl with ecstasy is likely to leave the next one limp with boredom. Sex researcher Shere Hite collected three thousand women's answers to her in-depth sex questionnaire, and her respondents' detailed descriptions of exactly how they get themselves off fill thirty-four fascinating pages of her now classic book *The Hite Report.* If you've never had an orgasm and you're looking for tips, check out the previous chapter.

Changing Your Self-Love Technique

SOMETIMES, WE HEAR from those who feel limited by their own masturbation technique. For instance, maybe you first orgasmed by lying in bed on your belly, squeezing your thigh muscles tight and pressing against your mattress. That technique may have worked fine when you were eleven, but as an adult you might find it limits your ability to have orgasms from other kinds of stimulation. If you want to be able to come from oral sex, or have an orgasm by rubbing your clit while you're enjoying penetration with a partner, the lying-on-your-belly-thigh-squeezing technique may present some challenges.

Similarly, some people with a penis get into the habit of waxing their pickle with a tightly clenched death grip. Human orifices aren't nearly as tight by comparison, which can make it challenging to have an orgasm during penetration with a partner. Varying your technique can make you a more versatile player between the sheets.

Good news: It's often possible to learn to masturbate and have orgasms in new ways. The process can be a little frustrating because you basically have to teach your body that it can respond to other kinds of stimulation—even when you know full well you could get off fast and easily your old way.

I couldn't get myself off with my hands for years, only with a vibrator. I finally taught myself when I was eighteen, and in the beginning it took a long time to orgasm. It was so frustrating and sometimes I'd quit before I came. Now I can get myself off with my hands in about five or six minutes and enjoy it a lot.

Magic of Ten Game

WANT TO HAVE stronger orgasms and be able to come in a wider variety of positions and situations? Here's a fun game you can play all by yourself that can help:

1. Wait until you have some private time.
2. Masturbate in your most common, reliable way. Get yourself almost to the brink of orgasm, but stop before you reach "the point of no return"—do *not* allow yourself to fall over that orgasmic edge. Count "one."
3. Change to a new position. If you were lying on your back, try kneeling on your bed, or sitting up with your back against the wall.

Start masturbating again. You will have lost some of your arousal but not all. Get yourself almost to the brink of orgasm again. It'll be a little more challenging this time because you're not accustomed to doing so in this position. Again, stop before you reach "the point of no return"—no orgasm allowed yet. That's "two."

4. Change to a new position. You might lie on your side, or crouch doggie style, resting on your knees and one forearm, using your head for support. You might try it with your legs closer together or farther apart than is your usual preference. Again, pleasure yourself almost to orgasm, but stop just before you get there. "Three."

5. Get yourself to that brink of orgasm ten times. You may find it helps to rest for a minute or two in between positions, to allow your level of arousal to fall back a bit before nudging it up again. On the tenth time, you're allowed to go for it—*finally*!

6. Enjoy an orgasm that will probably be particularly satisfying because of all that teasing. Longer buildups tend to result in bigger orgasms. Plus, realizing your body has the potential to come in so many different positions can be liberating!

For advanced players: Instead of just modifying your physical position, experiment with changing the type of stimulation each time. Try one finger instead of two, vertical strokes instead of horizontal, tapping instead of rubbing. Vary your typical speed or rhythm. Masturbate with various kinds of penetration, both fingers and other phallic objects. Warning: This is a lot harder, and some kinds of stimulation may not work for your body. That's okay—you can also alternate between your reliable way of touching yourself and new approaches. Make up the rules as you go. The best part of this game is that you discover a little more about how your body responds each time you play. There's no way to lose at a game that ends in orgasm!

To make this kind of change, start masturbating using your old technique. When you get pretty aroused, switch to a new technique that will allow you more orgasmic versatility. Stick with it even though it will take longer and may not feel as arousing right away—this may require some persistence. You'll probably need to experiment a bit to figure out what feels best and how to make this new technique work for you, much like someone who's learning to have an orgasm for the first time. (Your advantage is that you're starting with the confidence that comes with *knowing* your body is capable of having orgasms.) Make sure you orgasm using the new technique. If you're having trouble staying sufficiently aroused, switch back briefly to your old technique to boost your arousal, but then bring yourself to orgasm the new way. Keep practicing even though it'll take more time and might not feel like as much fun. Remember how many years you practiced your old technique, and be patient as your body learns this new way. (The resources we recommend on page 86 also have helpful suggestions on this subject.) Approach this like an experiment: if it works, great, and it's also fine if you decide to stick with your tried-and-true way of doing things.

Not Only for the Young

AT AGE EIGHTY-NINE, actress Gloria Stuart, who starred in films with everyone from Shirley Temple to Leonardo DiCaprio in *Titanic*, wrote in her autobiography, "I am devoted to masturbation. I think it's probably one of the most pleasurable things in my life. . . . I had, and have, no guilt whatsoever when it comes to pleasuring myself."

Paddling the Pink Canoe

WHY IS IT that there are about a hundred fun—if sometimes violent—slang phrases for masturbation involving a penis (jerking off, beating off, playing pocket pool, choking the chicken, spanking the monkey), but the English language leaves those of us with a clitoris so few choices? Luckily, self-pleasuring aficionados have been hard at work inventing and collecting slang for the rest of us. Next time, take your pick from many options:

beating around the bush
beating the beaver
bushwhacking

buttering the muffin
buzzing off
caressing the kitty

checking the oil
churning the butter
clitorizing
coaxing the genie out of the magic lamp
dipping fingers in the honey pot
double-clicking the mouse
fiddling the bean
finger dancing
flicking the switch
flitting my clit
getting to know myself
going pearl diving
going on a finger ride
having sex with someone I love
jilling off

letting my fingers do the walking
ménage à moi
paddling the pink canoe
parting the petals
petting the bunny
petting the pussy cat
plunging the happy hole
polishing the pearl
pushing the button
rowing the little man in the boat
rowing the little lady in the boat
rubbin' the nubbin
tiptoeing through the two-lips
two-finger tango
waxing the flesh taco

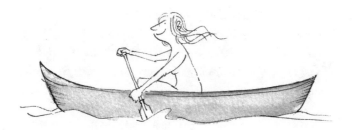

Masturbation for Trans Folks

A LOT OF trans and nonbinary people who haven't had genital surgeries like to think about masturbating in ways that aren't expected or typical for what their genitals look like. For example, a lot of trans masculine people will refer to masturbating as "jerking off," treating their dick the same way a cis guy would, even if it functions differently. Likewise, many trans femmes have found treating their penis as a large clitoris to be affirming and pleasurable, rubbing in circles and patterns, and finding rhythms that are exciting.

Some trans women and femmes have found a new form of fingering themselves (or getting fingered) called muffing. Essentially, muffing is fingering of the inguinal canal. This is the canal the testicles have descended from, and are useful for a lot of folks who tuck (moving the penis and testicles so that they're not visible in tight clothing). Within the scrotum, behind the testicles, are two canals that are about the diameter of your finger. Playing with them can be stimulating, but very sensitive to navigate. Check www.iloveorgasmsbook.com for more resources about muffing and sex for trans women in general.

Sex Tips for Partners

○ If your clitoris-owning partner masturbates, become this activity's number one fan. (Encourage them to support your solo sex too; this should go both ways.) Let your significant other know that you think it's great for a clitoris-owner to be good friends with their clit.

> *Until I was in a relationship, I hadn't discussed masturbation, aside from dirty jokes. My boyfriend considered masturbation (mine, at any rate) to be a positive thing and was eager to hear about what I liked. He provided me with enough encouragement to accept the practice of it, and do it more frequently.*

○ Encourage your partner to touch themselves while you're being sexual together if they're comfortable with this. (If they're not, they may warm up to the idea over time if you consistently let them know that *you're* comfortable with it.)

○ If your sweetie doesn't engage in solo sex, buy them a masturbation-positive book as a gift, and encourage them to read it. Or read it together! (Of course, if they don't want to masturbate or share their masturbatory adventures with you, you should respect their decision about something so personal.)

Making Online Sex Less Awkward

WHEN IT COMES to partnered sex, being able to touch each other is usually the whole point. But sometimes that's not possible, and thanks to technology the options for digital sex keep getting better.

But there's no question about it: Video sex, phone sex, and sexting can be cringey. Here are some ways to dial down the awkward and dial up the fun.

- **Consent and privacy first.** Talk about and respect each other's limits before you start. Don't screen record, screenshot, or share nudes or videos of someone without their permission. Unless you know and trust your partner incredibly well, consider not having your face and your genitals in the shot at the same time.
- **Send a teaser in advance.** Pique interest with a dirty text, a suggestive photo, or a few seconds of video earlier in the day.
- **Nudes don't have to be nude.** Sometimes less is more (less nakedness, more sexy, that is). It can feel more comfortable, and be just as provocative if not more, to wear something that makes you feel sexy rather than baring it all. Turning the lights down low or using candlelight can create ambience and make you feel less exposed than under the fluorescents.
- **Consider a phone holder.** For video chatting with a phone or tablet, a mount or stand can let you set it and forget it so you'll have your hands free and don't have to keep fidgeting with your device. Plus, it's easier to choose your favorite angle.
- **Masturbate.** Your partner's image or words alone are unlikely to bring you to orgasm—it's your own touch (or that of a vibrator or other sex toy) that can make digital sex superhot.
- **Go slow.** Foreplay is just as important for digital sex as for the in-person kind.
- **Tell your partner what you'd like to do with them if you were together.** If you're stuck for what to say, whispering what you'd like to do is always a great way to start. Take your time and let the scene you create together unfold slowly and sensuously.

○ **Or tell them how you're self-pleasuring.** Keep the camera on your face, and while you touch your own body, tell your partner exactly what you're doing and feeling with lots of details. Watching someone's face as they get aroused can be a real treat.

○ **Change up your angles, body parts, and locations.** Use pillows or your tripod to have video sex that is sometimes a close-up on your front, other times from behind. Emphasize your chest or your booty. Bring your device into the room while you take a bath—just make sure it stays dry!

○ **Invest in app-controlled sex toys.** One or both partners can have the power to "touch" the other with apps that let you pair up your toys (*teledildonics* is the fancy word) and boost the interactivity of your long-distance play. They're not cheap, though.

○ **Consider voice only or text only.** Since video chat is instantly accessible it can feel obvious to start there. But sometimes old-fashioned phone sex is less awkward and just as sexy. Ditto for sexting with words or photos only, video free. Especially if you find yourself self-conscious on camera or are concerned about a partner you don't know well screen-recording your video, sticking with voice or text can be liberating. The goal is to relax and enjoy, and sometimes that's way easier with your camera *off*.

4

Going Down, Down, Baby
Oral Sex and Orgasm

Let's talk about tongue-on-clitoris. It's a beloved combination for many vulva-owners, an exquisitely pleasurable combination of body parts. Likewise for penis-owners, mouth-on-penis is similarly beloved. For many, the combination of mouth, tongue, and lips is uniquely delightful.

Of the two, cunnilingus is more fraught with misgivings, uncertainties, and questions for both vulva-owners and their partners. So, while this chapter includes some advice for improving your blow job game, it will center on pussy-eating, muff-diving, yodeling in the valley.

When "tongues" first come up in our programs as a possible source of orgasms, audiences frequently cheer. Why so popular? Well, tongues are wet, soft, and warm, fast or slow, and they can make all sorts of luscious strokes. In short, they're brilliantly designed for clitoral stimulation, the anatomical heart of orgasm for most people with a vulva. In our survey, we asked vulva-owners their favorite way to have an orgasm, and 20 percent of them said oral sex, second only to the 25 percent who said their fave was intercourse combined with clitoral stimulation. Certainly, not everyone likes to receive oral sex, and not all partners want to give it, but for many, oral action is one of sex's sweetest delicacies.

Cunnilingus wasn't always an "everybody's doing it" sort of activity in the

United States. For the generation born in the 1930s, oral sex wasn't something "good husbands and wives" (and certainly not unmarried/dating couples) did— only about 44 percent of women in that generation had received oral sex in their lifetime (or admitted it to researchers who asked). Many baby boomers say that in their day, oral sex was considered far more intimate than intercourse, something some couples would do only if they felt truly comfortable with each other. Still, they did do it, and the numbers climbed. Nowadays, 87 percent of all people aged 25 to 70+ have received oral sex. The numbers aren't quite as high yet among 18- to 24-year-olds, but it seems likely they'll catch up—some haven't yet found a partner to take a trip downtown.

Why is it so popular? It feels good!

The first time I had an orgasm was when my boyfriend at the time gave me oral stimulation. It was amazing. I told him that if he wanted to he could do that every hour on the hour for the rest of my life.

A lot of partners are pretty enthusiastic too:

I think it's wild that I can drive someone to orgasm just with my mouth. I love the variety of light touch to mild bites, from intense pressure with my tongue to even my warm breath nearby but not touching any skin. Mix that with taste, smell, and having legs wrapped around my head and I'm there!

It's lots of fun to be able to pleasure a woman while being so close to the center of pleasure. I also think there's beauty in the female genitalia. It's great to be able to not worry about yourself and focus completely on her pleasure.

At first I just wanted to try going down on her. Her reaction and mood afterward make me want me to do it over and over again. It's the only thing I can do that makes her cry out my name and use the phrase, "Oh, God."

Despite the popularity of oral sex, it brings up a *lot* of mixed feelings. Some people aren't receiving as much as they'd like. Some are too self-conscious, some have partners who don't like to give oral sex, and some aren't sure how to ask for more.

Is Oral on the Agenda?

WE ASKED OUR survey respondents with a vulva whether their partner performed oral sex on them in their most recent partnered sexual experience. Here's what they said.

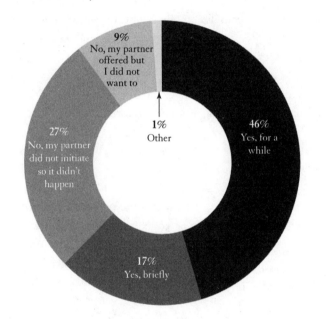

9%
No, my partner offered but I did not want to

27%
No, my partner did not initiate so it didn't happen

1%
Other

46%
Yes, for a while

17%
Yes, briefly

People who checked "Other" said they had their period, preferred being stroked by their partner's finger, had been feeling too insecure for oral sex, and so on.

Oral sex on men is so external whereas on women it's so internal and much more personal. You could give a man head while he still has his pants on! But for a woman, you have to be right there, between her legs, and she has to open up (literally and figuratively) and give herself to you.

I think I'm too shy about asking for oral sex. I enjoy spontaneity, but I would be lying if I said I didn't want it more. I need to speak up and ask for it more often.

My girlfriend won't perform oral sex on me very often (she's only done it about three times) because she's sensitive to my smell and taste. I don't mind doing it to her, but it sucks for me.

Oral sex can bring up complex emotions for transgender and nonbinary people too. On the one hand (on the one tongue?), mouths and tongues plus genitals is a winning combination for lots of people. But on the other, to perform oral sex your partner is literally putting their face directly in front of and up against your genitals. For someone who doesn't have the best relationship with their genitals, it's understandable that they might not be comfortable receiving oral.

I don't like oral sex because of my dysphoria. I've never gotten off that way. Do only what makes you feel comfortable and don't be ashamed of what you do like.

Cunnilingus Is Nothing New

ORAL SEX'S POPULARITY has grown tremendously, but it's not a new invention. The Kama Sutra, written as early as 400 BCE, features it, as does ancient erotic art in Japan and China.

Although some people find other kinds of sex more or equally pleasurable, many of our survey respondents of all gender identities expressed a desire to make oral sex a bigger part of their lives. Since feeling self-conscious about receiving it or about asking for it was a major barrier for many, let's dive into that issue first. If you're already an oral sex enthusiast, skip right down to the positions on page 128.

How to Blow the Love Whistle (a.k.a. the Penis)

THIS CHAPTER CENTERS oral sex on vulvas because this book's primary goal is to provide orgasm assistance to those who need it the most. Most of the advice here focuses on the needs of vulva-owners and their partners, because based on our conversations with penis-owners, they simply aren't wrestling with the same levels of self-consciousness and self-doubt about receiving oral sex. However, there are still some questions of technique that may be helpful to those who choose to lick the lollipop.

We asked penis-owners for their top advice to partners who want to give a great blow job, and overall we were struck by the straightforward simplicity of their recommendations. "Traditional" advice from experts is usually filled with complex step-by-step choreography: swirl the tongue here, cup the balls this way, try this trick for deep throating without gagging. By comparison, the overwhelming response from penis-owners boiled down to these six top tips:

1. For crying out loud, please do everything you can to keep your teeth away from my dick!
2. Use your hands, not just your mouth.
3. Focus most of your attention on the head.
4. Use plenty of saliva to be sure it's good and wet down there.
5. Play with the balls a bit too. (A small percentage said, "Leave my balls alone," so check in about this one.)
6. Lots of extra points for enthusiasm and enjoyment.

Imagine it's the most delicious popsicle you've ever had.

You know what they say: If you love what you do, it shows. Really slurp and get messy, and don't be afraid to use your hands.

Basically, hundreds of people with a penis, unaware of what the others had submitted, gave exactly the same advice. Here are a few more things from our results that might surprise you:

Deep throating barely registered. Literally only 1 percent of respondents mentioned deep throating. We suspect a lot of blow job–givers worry about how to deep throat or feel like failures if they can't do so comfortably. Our advice: Don't worry about it! Use your hand (see top tip #2) on the shaft, wet with saliva (see top tip #4), as an extension of your mouth to stimulate the shaft. Boom. You've transformed your "mouth" into a long, wet tube, and the penis no longer needs to go down your throat. Aiming the phallus into your cheek (rather than down your throat) can help too.

"Slower" and "rhythmic" were recommended often. As a group, our survey takers recommended slower blow jobs rather than faster, some emphasizing the importance of starting slow. Many talked about pacing yourself, being consistent, and finding a rhythm. We wonder if the "fast and furious blow job" is yet another example of a way that porn can be misleading.

Take your time. Going faster isn't always better.

For every rule, there's an exception. While "no teeth" was top advice, 1 percent requested "light teeth." While many respondents mentioned enjoying a bit of attention to their balls, 1 percent said no, it's better to leave their scrotum alone. Although "use your hand!" was popular guidance, 4 percent asked caring fellators to minimize use of their hand or not use it at all. Many, many survey takers advised partners to communicate, ask for feedback, and listen to the penis-owner's sounds and breathing to guide them.

Don't try to replicate what you see in porn, just do what you can and have fun with it. Ask your partner if something feels good or if they like certain motions.

It's hard to do it wrong. Just pay attention to your partner's breath and you'll learn what they like.

A little eye contact is hot.

Asking for feedback is definitely "golden rule" advice—in our own experience, most partners of *all* genders would prefer a partner who checks in, asks questions, and listens rather than one who assumes that you like sex exactly the way their last partner did. Checking in (especially with a mouth full of cock) can be challenging, to put it mildly. You might find some of the tips in Chapter 8 helpful.

Overall, the advice was collectively best summed up by this one, fortune cookie–worthy survey comment: "As long as there is effort, I will be satisfied."

Spit or Swallow?

THE ANSWER: IT'S really up to the blow job giver. Do penis-owners think it's cool if their partners swallow? According to our survey, yes, many do. But we think it's fair to say that nearly all would *much* prefer to receive a blow job that ends in a quiet spit into a tissue than not to receive a blow job at all. So, if swallowing isn't a big deal to you, then sure, swallow. But if you'd rather not, have the tissue box nearby and don't worry about it.

A third path to consider is using a condom for oral sex, maybe even a flavored one (that's why they exist). According to one national study of over 2,100 adults, 10 percent said they always or often used a condom or dental dam for oral sex. Rates were similar for married, single, and partnered people.

Flavored condoms have expanded beyond banana and strawberry—now you can get ultrathin condoms in flavors like chocolate, vanilla, mint, piña colada, and tequila sunrise. Here are some Amazon reviews to give you a sense:

After 34 years I finally got my first one because of these—THANK YOU! She said it tasted good and that she would "do it again":):):)

Wife enjoyed these almost as much as I did. She said it does have an aftertaste but is a million times better than the flavor of the finish without them. We have ordered more for the fun to continue.

Or if you're not into the flavors, just choose an unlubricated condom (oral sex is why they exist too). You can even search "tasteless condoms" for the top picks in non-rubbery-tasting prophylactics. (Skyn condoms are getting excellent reviews as this goes to print.)

Not only will a condom eliminate the spit-or-swallow conundrum, oral sex *can* transmit STIs. Using a condom dramatically reduces your risk.

Receiving Lip Service: Overcoming Shyness and Self-Consciousness

UNLESS YOU'RE A contortionist or a superbly flexible gymnast, oral sex offers your partner a closer view of your vulva than you could ever get of your own. And it's not just the view: Partners get to touch, smell, and taste. Some people with a vulva squirm uncomfortably at the very thought of what the experience might be like "down there" for a partner. As one woman wrote on our survey, "It's dark!"

We asked our vulva-owning survey respondents who haven't received all that much oral sex in their lives the reasons why. The number one response, with 43 percent of respondents naming it, was being uncomfortable with how their genitals look, smell, or taste. It's not surprising that many vulva-owners are shy, if not profoundly uneasy, about letting a partner get too close to their private parts. Our culture doesn't offer much support in the vulva self-esteem department. As we've discussed earlier, many grew up surrounded by messages that their genitals are dirty and shameful. Middle school slang describes vulvas and vaginas as smelly and expressions like "carpet munching" make oral sex on a vulva sound about as appealing as chewing on a doormat. Douche commercials sell the idea that vulvas need products to make them smell better, planting more suspicion that the Y is an unpleasant place to dine. The few places where people get to see what vulvas look like—porn and textbook line drawings—generally fail to show the vibrant diversity of colors, shapes, and sizes that are healthy and normal.

In reality, most vulva-owners who are terrified of how they taste or smell are basing their feelings on fear rather than experience. If this describes you, you can do a reality check: Put your finger down there, bring it up to your nose and mouth, and experience it for yourself.

I tasted my own stuff, just to see what I was subjecting others to, and realized it's not bad at all!

Va-jay-jays do have their own smell that's unique to each person, just like the variation in the scents of lovers' skin, hair, mouth, and penises. But the smell of a vulva isn't necessarily a bad one—in fact, a lot of people say it grew on them over time. The pH of a healthy vagina is about the same as a glass of red wine, and like wine, it can be an acquired taste. Many report that their feelings about their taste or smell changed when they saw a partner unbothered by it—or totally turned on. Indeed, several research studies reported that most partners say it's pleasurable to go down on a vulva.

I was so scared the first time. And I still am now. I constantly asked—or rather bugged—my partner whether he liked what he was doing. Or if he was sure. Although I wanted him to do it very much, I was scared that I was too smelly there. I asked him if he was doing it for my pleasure alone, or if he enjoyed it as well, and he reassured me that he loved it, and, in fact, it smelled great and tasted great. I don't think I fully believe him yet!

As a lesbian, every vulva tastes different! And they are all equally beautiful.

I had concerns until my current partner assured me that he loved the way I looked, smelled, and tasted, and that he loved giving me oral sex. Then I stopped being self-conscious and just let myself feel good.

Vulvas can taste and smell different at different times during the menstrual cycle. Partners may notice differences just before their partner's period, just after it, and around ovulation (unless they use hormonal birth control). You might see whether there are times of the month your partner particularly enjoys your taste or would prefer to avoid, and plan your oral interludes accordingly. Also, though vulvas do taste different from one another and people frequently come up with theories about how this is affected by what they eat or drink, most people who *try* to change their taste by eating large amounts of some food (pineapple is the most famous one) haven't found much, if any, change. Many partners have commented, however, that smokers have a noticeably bitter taste.

Will Pineapple Make Me Taste Better?

HOW TO MAKE your bodily fluids taste better is a question we get from both people with a vulva and those with a penis. The answer is the same for all genders. See pages 116–117.

Or maybe it's your vulva's physical appearance that stresses you out? Keep in mind that when it comes to vulvas and vaginas, "normal" is a *very* wide range. Whatever color, shape, or size you've got, symmetrical or not, most likely it's more common than you realize. As one person wrote on our survey, "I would just like to remind you that anyone having sex with you already thinks you're hot!"

One reason for many people's insecurity is that they remember what their own genitals looked like when they were a kid. Maybe no one told you that as other body parts change during puberty—pubic hair, breasts, and all the rest—vulvas change too. As an adult, it's normal to have one or both "inner lips" protrude outside the "outer lips" (who named them that, anyway?). Your "new look" doesn't mean something went wrong, simply that your body is no longer a child's body. As adults, we have curves *all over*. Befriend Your Vulva, page 60, may help you make peace with your nether regions.

It is a requirement for my sexual partner to feel comfortable with my body, otherwise they have no business being this close to me.

What about period sex?

WHEN PEOPLE ASK about having sex during a period, usually they're thinking about penetrative sex. But what about oral sex? Either kind is fine to have if both partners want to! And there are potential benefits since orgasms can relieve menstrual cramps. It's important to be aware that blood can transmit viruses like HIV and hepatitis B.

Oral sex during that phase of the moon doesn't necessarily mean blood on the face. Many couples find blood is minimal to nonexistent if it's a light flow day and the person who has their period takes a quick shower in advance. Some people with a vagina like to insert a menstrual cup or disk before they shower, basically an alternative to pads or tampons that catches the period blood up high, against the cervix. Some menstrual cups are even designed to sit far enough inside the vagina that penetrative sex works too.

Tips for Boosting Your Oral Sex Self-Esteem

1. Shower before sex. Showering before a date or before you expect to be in a sexual situation is generally good etiquette, given that most people aren't fans of armpit odor either. That said, many people are far more worried about the way their own body smells than they need to be, and most couples don't feel the need to run to the shower every time sex is on the horizon. Among the many benefits of having a partner you trust and have built a rapport with is that you can rely on each other to suggest a quick break for both of you to brush your teeth or hop into the shower together. Also, be aware that there are plenty of people who find the naturally heady, musky scents of a sweaty, unwashed body to be an incredible turn-on. Know thy partner!

I do feel better about receiving oral sex after I shower or when I'm feeling very fresh and clean. I want to be clean and tasty for my partner, so sometimes I suggest a shower as foreplay. That way we're both clean and we get to spend time together naked before we're actually in bed. And sometimes we never make it to bed!

What Your History Books Didn't Mention About Napoléon

YOU MAY VAGUELY remember learning in high school history class about French emperor and military leader Napoléon Bonaparte. What your history teacher probably didn't mention (and probably didn't know themselves) was that Napoléon was "obsessed by cunnilingus" and talked about it frequently, according to historian and biographer Andrew Roberts. Roberts reports that, in letters to his first wife, Napoléon would say, "Don't wash for three days" because he'd enjoy going down on her when she was unwashed.

2. Stay clean in vagina-friendly ways. A typical vagina is slightly acidic on the pH scale (and you thought that chemistry class would be irrelevant to your life!), which helps it fight disease-causing bacteria and keep cervical cells healthy. Soap, on the other hand, is alkaline, so washing inside a vagina with soap throws off the balance and can even make it smell worse. Vaginas clean themselves constantly, sort of like eyes—both are generally better off if you let them do their own thing and only wash around the outside. All the vagina-owner needs to do is rinse the vulva (the outside parts) and entrance to the vagina gently with warm water. If you feel you absolutely must use soap, choose something very mild, without dyes or perfumes, or a soap that advertises itself as having a low pH.

Along the same lines, vaginas definitely do not like douching (spraying water or fluids into them). Unless you have a medical problem for which douching is a treatment, skip it. Douches disturb the normal pH levels and can spread infections, potentially leading to pelvic inflammatory disease or bacterial vaginosis. Your vagina wasn't designed to smell like a plug-in air freshener, and your partner isn't expecting it to.

I clean myself every time before sex…just with water, washcloth, and a mild unscented soap. I used to be big into using perfumes and smelly soap, but I learned to be natural.

3. Consider a latex barrier. In addition to reducing the risk of HIV and STI transmission, barriers like dental dams are also an excellent way to reduce taste and smell. These issues matter a great deal to some and not at all to others. But if you're feeling self-conscious, your partner is having a hard time coping, or you have your period, a dental dam can be a great option to allow you to focus on pleasure without getting hung up on taste, smell, or appearance.

Silky latex panties are another option: A company called Lorals (a play on "love oral always") sells ultrathin ones designed for oral sex and rimming. We find particularly ingenious their marketing of the many ways they can be used: curbing the discomfort of a partner's facial hair, protecting sheets from period blood, and even simply playing with them as a form of kinky underwear ("snap, stretch, or rip through our slinky latex to kink things up").

Of course, there are lower-cost barriers too. Plastic wrap, available in just about every kitchen in the country, also blocks out tastes and smells. A nice, long sheet of plastic wrap may be just what you need to reap the benefits of an enthusiastic tongue while sidestepping the issue of taste and smell. If you wrap it right, it will stick to itself, allowing for hands-free fun. For added sensation, add a few drops of lube on the vulva side of a dental dam or sheet of plastic wrap.

4. Get beyond the awkwardness. Do you identify with these comments?

For a while I wouldn't let my partner give me oral sex. I felt all vulnerable lying there naked alone while he was off exploring part of me that I wasn't comfortable with yet myself.

I've felt nervous and uncomfortable to the point of pushing guys away and saying, "Oh, you don't have to do that." They take what I say to mean that I don't want them to, or probably that they're doing a bad job. Then everyone just gets humiliated and uncomfortable. Really, I guess I'm probably hoping they'll say, "No, I really want to," and keep at it. Maybe it's all just a process of looking for confirmation that in fact I'm not gross, smelly, taking too long, etc.

I don't like partners to give me oral sex with bright lights on, and sometimes I put my hands on my stomach, because I feel chubby.

If you recognize these thoughts and emotions, you're definitely not alone. Here are some things to try:

○ **Think about how early sexual experiences may have affected you.** How your first few partners treated you and reacted to your body can have a huge impact, particularly if they said negative or disparaging things since you had no basis for comparison yet. Experiences like sexual abuse or assault can add to the challenges.

> *The first person who ever went down on me told me that I smelled funny and tasted funny. It took me a long time to get over feeling self-conscious as a result of that experience. Luckily I had another partner who told me how much he loved how I tasted and smelled and was so enthusiastic*

about giving me oral sex that I was able to start feeling sexy about receiving it.

If a past partner has been critical of your body, remind yourself that their comments were rude, and that many partners are likely to feel very differently!

○ **Don't expect perfection.** Remember that sex in the real world will never be the picture-perfect acts and bodies you see in porn or on TV. In sex on the screen and in romance novels, no one ever farts or queefs (that's when air "farts" out the vagina—charming!), people never accidentally elbow their partners in the head while changing positions, and no one ever has to pause to extract a pubic hair from their teeth. In real life, these things happen. No biggie. You're not expected to be perfection on wheels in bed.

Honestly, getting older and gaining more confidence in who I am as a human helped. At this point in my life, I'm like "Well, dick isn't pretty or tasty either, so go down to town or get the heck out."

○ **Fake it until you make it.** We don't recommend faking orgasms, but by faking confidence and comfort—maybe even pretending to be someone whose sexual self-confidence you admire—you might actually internalize that confidence over time.

The dude (I've only had sex with men/people with a penis) is just happy to be there, so I don't stress about it. There's a positive feedback cycle of me moaning while receiving oral, them getting more into it, me getting wetter and moaning more, then getting even more into it until orgasm happens. So faking it helps???

I've learned to be more confident and proud of my body. I've realized that a lot of the concerns I had aren't shared by my partners! Sex can be fun, great, fantastic, mind-blowing even. It can also be messy, smelly, sweaty, and awkward. Relax and go with it! It's worth it in the end, right?

5. It's okay to say no. You don't have to like oral sex. If you're just not that into it, it's fine to say, "No, thanks." Your feelings may change over time as you become more experienced sexually or have different partners with different attitudes or techniques. Or they may not, and that's totally okay too. Oral sex is one option among many, and there are plenty of people who prefer other activities instead.

It's a really intimate experience that I don't share with a lot of people. Sometimes I'd rather have my partner where I can make eye contact and hold/kiss.

6. Ask for it. The flip side of "It's okay to say no" is "It's okay to ask for what you want!" Asking for something sexual can take courage, but it usually works to your advantage (this goes for every sexual act under the sun, not just oral sex). Think about it:

○ The worst-case scenario is that you ask, and your partner says they'd rather not. Although that would be disappointing, you haven't lost any ground; you ended up just where you started out.

○ Think about times your partner has asked you for something sexually and you agreed. There's a good chance you enjoyed getting your partner off or intensifying their pleasure. Or perhaps your partner shares your interest in oral sex but is too shy to go for it, too insecure about their skills, or unsure about how to bring it up.

○ Partners aren't mind readers. Unless you've discussed the issue before, it's unfair to assume that your partner doesn't go down on you because they dislike it. It's possible your partner forgot about it because they're doing things "the usual way," or don't realize how much you enjoy it.

> ## When to Call the Doc
>
> GET YOUR VAGINA checked out by your health-care provider or a local health clinic if it has:
>
> - A distinctly bad odor that doesn't go away
>
> - An unusual vaginal discharge (All vaginas have normal vaginal secretions that change throughout the menstrual cycle—you want to pay attention to something that's different or smells particularly bad.)
>
> - An itching or burning sensation
>
> These could be the symptoms of a yeast infection, an STI, or something else that requires medical attention. Some clinics, including many Planned Parenthood centers, provide services on a sliding scale based on income.

○ Just as you have the right to ask, your partner has the right to say no or make a modified proposal ("How about we do that this weekend when we both have time to shower first?"). Asking isn't forcing your partner to do something they don't want to do.

I know my girlfriend won't go down on me unless she wants to. And if she's not enjoying it, she'll stop and use her hands—which is fine with me. It's good to know she doesn't feel like she has to.

If someone doesn't want to go down on you, it's their problem. But don't let the fear of that stop you from asking for what you need to be pleased.

If you're trying to find the right words to ask, here are some to try on for size:

○ *How about we trade? I'll do you, you do me.*
○ *How do you feel about going down on your partners? It's one of my favorite things.*
○ *We haven't done oral sex on me in a while—would you be up for it?*
○ *I was just thinking about that other time when you ate me out—that orgasm was incredible. Would you be in the mood to do it again?*
○ *I'd love it if you'd go down on me.*

Gender-Affirming Options

LOTS OF TRANS and nonbinary people do their best to craft strategies that work (most of the time) for them: only agreeing to oral with a partner they trust and with whom they communicate well, choosing affirming words for their genitals or the act (even in their own mind), engaging in oral sex only on days when they have the emotional capacity, practicing self-love, and so on. For some, hormones and/or surgery that bring about physical changes improve both their mental and emotional well-being and their experience of oral sex.

It gives me dysphoria, especially in positions where I'm straddling. I like using more gender-affirming language for it, but I really have to be in a certain mood.

For a long time I had anxiety because I was afraid my pussy didn't look like an AFAB [assigned female at birth] pussy should look like. Now my balls just give me euphoria. I like to use terms like "blowjob" instead of "eating out" or something.

I love my bottom growth and it added a lot of confidence for me. Before I was really insecure, but after I have little to no insecurity about it.

69: The Fantasy (Usually) Exceeds the Reality

SIXTY-NINE IS ONE of the most famous numbers on earth because it's the slang name for the act of two people simultaneously performing oral sex on each other. The numbers sort of represent the shapes of the two bodies facing each other side by side, one right-side up, one upside down. The appeal, of course, is the potential to receive pleasure at the same time, not usually possible with oral sex. Plus, 69 keeps you close together, making it perhaps a more intimate position than most approaches to oral sex.

We'd never heard of anyone doing a 69 survey before, but we figured the time was long overdue. Our findings confirmed our suspicions:

○ Most people have tried it (or want to).
○ Most people (though certainly not all) conclude that it's better in theory than in practice.

Sixty-nine is the ultimate in multitasking. Sex educators Em and Lo put it best when they wrote, "Developing a rhythm [during 69] requires the coordination of a Cirque du Soleil performer, the patience of a Buddhist monk, and the motor skills of a bonobo ape. To say nothing of the concentration skills required." Here's what typical 69 critics had to say on our survey:

I'm afraid if he does something that feels particularly good, I'll accidentally bite him.

I hate 69. It's physically awkward (I'm very petite and my partners have generally been very tall) and I find it too distracting. I'm working too hard at what I'm doing to enjoy what I'm getting, but I can't entirely ignore what I'm getting in order to focus 100 percent on what I'm doing!

It's difficult to say, "Harder," or "Gentler," or "Up a bit" when one has a mouthful of cock.

But the act does have its share of fans. Penis-owners seem to be a bit more enthusiastic about 69 than vulva-owners overall, perhaps because those with a vulva are more likely to find they need honed concentration to be able to have an orgasm. These comments are all from vulva-owners in the pro-69 camp, though:

Most of the time I like it because I like how my partner's pleasure contributes to my pleasure and vice versa. The first time I ever experienced simultaneous orgasm with a partner was in this position.

I love it! I like it because it prevents me from fully concentrating on myself and what's happening between my legs—it's distracting in a good way. I also really like giving head—it turns me on and turning on a partner is really hot. Sometimes it can be frustrating if my partner stops giving me head because it gets too distracting for him. I come more easily from this than anything except masturbation, I think.

I've tried it before with men, and with the female partner I'm currently with. With men, it's pretty awkward if the woman is ever on the bottom because she has a hard time controlling how far the penis is going into her mouth. Doing the 69 position with another woman is absolutely amazing. It allows one to grind and to sort of tease. INCREDIBLE!

If you're going to try it, keep in mind that there are two possible positions for 69-ing: side by side and top/bottom. In the top/bottom position, many people whose partner has a penis have strong opinions about whether they prefer to be on the bottom (where they can relax) or on top (where they can control how deeply their partner's penis goes into their mouth). Side by side, both partners can relax more, and there's less of a feeling of having your partner's anus too close to your nose, but the angle of stimulation can be trickier.

Think-outside-the-box 69-ers point out there's no law that says both people have to use their mouths the whole time. Some prefer modifications where the two partners take turns, alternating their oral attentions back and forth, or where one person uses manual stimulation while the other does oral. For instance, some find it easier to give a hand job or hold a vibrator for their partner while they receive oral sex, which gives the partner a chance to receive more genital pleasure than they normally would while going down.

Oral Sex Tips for Partners (How to Be a Cunning Linguist)

THE PREREQUISITES TO giving great oral sex are a positive attitude, a willingness to try and to learn, and a reasonable amount of patience. If you've got all three, you're well along the treasure trail already. Let's take a closer look:

1. A positive attitude. More important than whether your tongue flicks side to side, up and down, or turns backflips is whether your partner gets the sense that you enjoy—or at least are *absolutely* comfortable with—going down. If you get suited up with goggles and a snorkel, we guarantee your partner won't let you stay down there for long (and definitely won't be having any orgasms). Among our survey respondents who haven't received much oral sex, 37 percent said their partner's lack of enthusiasm was one of the reasons why. The number one thing that helps your partner relax, which needs to happen to enjoy what you're doing down there, is knowing that you want to give pleasure this way, don't see this as punishment, and maybe even (gasp!) enjoy it yourself. If you like licking between the labia, by all means let your partner know. If it turns you on, don't keep that a

Positions for Going Lips to Lips

POSITION	HOW IT WORKS	BENEFITS
Classic R & R (Rest and Recline)	Receiver lies on back or reclines against pillows, giver lies or kneels between legs.	■ Receiver can relax, close their eyes, and focus on the pleasure radiating from below. ■ Easy access to vulva, clit, and vagina for giver.
Edge-o'-the-Bed	Receiver sits or lies on bed, slides crotch to the edge of the bed. Giver kneels on the floor or sits on a low stool beside the bed.	■ Less neck strain for the giver than the Classic R&R position. ■ Easy access for giver. Great for using fingers or toys.
Throne (a.k.a. Royal Highness)	Receiver slouches in an armchair, couch, or seat with padded back, giver sits on floor or footstool.	■ Easier for partners to see each other since both are partly upright. ■ Easy access for giver.
Sitting on Face (variation: Cooler Sex)	Partner lies flat on back, vulva-owner kneels over them, positioning vulva over mouth.	■ Receiver has some control over pressure and location of stimulation by moving hips and raising/lowering self slightly. ■ Some givers find this position particularly sexy and like the view up at their partner. ■ Giver can lie back and relax.

DRAWBACKS	TIPS
■ Can lead to stiff neck and back pain for giver, especially if they stay put for a while.	■ Use pillows under the butt and/or under giver's chest to improve the angle.
■ Not much body contact between partners—can feel far away from each other.	■ Don't spread your legs too wide unless you want to (that's a porn technique designed to maximize visibility, not usually preferred in real life).
■ Where to put your legs? Dangling them off the bed isn't comfortable for long.	■ Try having the receiver rest their feet on the giver's back or shoulders, on the mattress, or on other things (chairs or boxes) you set up.
■ Might require a trip to Ikea to find the perfect chair.	■ Use pillows to adjust both partners' heights.
■ Some receivers find it comfortable to rest their feet on the floor or on the chair; others experience the leg-dangling problem.	■ If you push the chair up to the bed, you can put your feet on the bed.
	■ If you don't want a wet spot on your nicest armchair, put down a sheet or towel before settling in.
■ Some people get tired supporting their weight up there, find it difficult to relax enough for arousal to build.	■ Use pillows under giver's head to raise it, so receiver's legs don't have to be spread so wide.
■ Position makes some feel self-conscious.	■ Major improvement: Give receiver something to lean on, like a headboard or something sold as sex furniture. Budget option: put a big sturdy cooler (the kind you use to keep the drinks cold for a picnic or tailgate party) on the bed, covered with a sheet or towel and pillows.
■ Some givers feel uncomfortable about having less control and reduced ability to "come up for air."	

POSITION	HOW IT WORKS	BENEFITS
Thigh Pillow	Both people lie on their sides, perpendicular to each other. Receiver lifts top leg, and giver rests head on the inner thigh of lower leg.	■ Relaxing for both partners. ■ Nice body contact. ■ Face perpendicular to vulva allows for different angles of stimulation than most other positions, which are straight on.
On Your Knees	Receiver stands, giver kneels in front.	■ A classic position for cis guys to receive head (some blow job givers think it's hot, others find it degrading). Penis-owners aren't the only ones who can enjoy this position, though, and some people with a vulva like it precisely because it's often a "guy's position." ■ Can be done spontaneously in small spaces and "naughty" places.
Specialty Furniture	Google "sex furniture" to find a multitude of companies selling inspiring furniture designed to expand on sex position options.	■ Who isn't intrigued by the idea of furniture designed specifically for sex? ■ Can be used for intercourse, anal sex, and other sexual activities too. ■ Invaluable for some people whose back, knee, hip problems, or disabilities limit their sex position options.

DRAWBACKS	TIPS
■ Can be trickier to get the right stimulation. Fewer options since neither partner can move much. ■ What to do with the top leg?	■ Experiment with facing the same direction or facing opposite directions.
■ Many receivers get tired of standing after a while and want to sit or lie down to fully appreciate the sensations. ■ Hard on the knees of the kneeler.	■ Receiver will probably feel more stable if they stand with their back against a wall. ■ Use a pillow under the giver's knees if they want to go at it for a while but still walk later. ■ Consider starting out this way, then moving to another position to finish.
■ Expensive! ■ You can't return it if you try it out and decide you don't like it. ■ Where to store it when it's not in use?	■ If you're willing to be creative, you can probably find cheaper alternatives with firm pillows and furniture around the house. Plus, flea markets and garage sales have never been so much fun as when you're shopping for a footstool of just the right height.

secret. If you think the color or shape of your partner's vulva is beautiful, say so. And if you enjoy your partner's taste or scent, or just the way you can feel or hear the pleasure running through your partner's body, say so!

My partner assured me that he liked the taste and smell. We also explored the way it looked together with a mirror. Doing that really helped me feel at ease about myself and helped us bond.

That doesn't mean you should lie if these things *aren't* true for you—most people have pretty good BS meters, and if your partner gets the sense you're feeding falsehoods, that could backfire big time. If taste or smell is a challenge for you, check out some of the tips earlier in this chapter.

If you have some less-than-positive opinions on the subject, follow the adage about "if you can't say something nice," and keep that opinion to yourself. We're struck by how many people with a vulva struggle to recover from comments made by a partner, even many years earlier:

In theory I know my vagina is normal. But my partner said once ten years ago that they didn't like the way I taste and I think about it every time we have sex.

I was married for a long time to someone who had an aversion to female genitalia (sight, smells, taste), and this affected me negatively for many years. I became extremely self-conscious and began to view my genitals the same way they did: as bad and undesirable. Since ending that relationship, I have worked hard to fall back in love with my own body.

2. **A willingness to try and to learn.** This is easy enough: You let your partner know that you're willing, you initiate oral sex sometimes, you experiment and ask for tips and feedback. This doesn't mean you go down if your partner doesn't want you to. But your positive attitude makes a huge difference here. On our survey, one of the most common pieces of advice people with a vulva gave about oral sex was to pay closer attention to cues like moans, movements, and suggestions.

Facial Hair Alert

PARTNERS WITH BEARDS and stubble, take note! Beards are usually soft. But a day or two of stubble, and sometimes freshly cut beards, can cause "beard burn" and "stache rash" when they rub against a partner's face or between their thighs. That's because the tips of the hairs are sharper when they're freshly cut. This seems to be a risk especially for bare skin—a cushion of pubic hair can be excellent protection against hair-inflicted injuries. That said, your partner might adore your stubble! Be aware of the risks, and check in. In general, an "older" (not freshly cut) beard or a fresh shave are the most skin-friendly options.

Tell your partner before you begin, "I want you to tell me what you need. Tell me if you want faster or slower, etc." If a partner does this in a serious tone, the woman is likely to feel safe and comfortable giving instructions.

Make it all about the girl, listen to her body language and you'll know what she likes. Moans and hip movements mean that she wants more. So give it to her!

To be fair, the person receiving oral sex should remember to let their partner know how it feels, to avoid the problem this partner described:

I usually feel very unsure about "how things are going" while I'm performing oral sex, whether the act has become monotonous or if the woman is enjoying it. I often feel like I have no idea if I'm actually producing pleasure.

3. A reasonable amount of patience. As you know, on average it takes a person with a vulva longer to have an orgasm than a person with a penis. Penis-in-vagina sex leaves many penis-owners struggling against fate, doing everything in their power not to come too quickly. Cunnilingus doesn't have that same pressure—theoretically, it can last until the receiving partner is satisfied, as long as the giving partner still has the strength to lift their tongue.

This removes one pressure but creates a new one. The giving partner may be eager to get their own turn at receiving pleasure, not only giving it. (Although some people find giving oral sex totally sexy, it's a rare partner who can get off this way without some added genital stimulation.) Some partners are notorious for paying lip service to oral sex but ultimately not spending enough time down there. A few licks of the clit, and *BAM!*—back up, ready for intercourse or something else that will give *them* an orgasm.

The simple awareness that orgasms through oral can take a while can lead some vulva-owners to take a pass. Among our survey respondents who haven't received much oral sex, 28 percent said they were concerned about how long it takes.

People with a vulva repeatedly say that their favorite cunning linguists are the ones who make clear they're willing to spend as much time as the oral recipient needs. This message can be communicated in gentle reassurances ("I'm in no rush," "We've got lots of time," "I'm happy to keep going as long as you want"). Or it can be communicated nonverbally, with enthusiastic oral sex until the vulva-owner comes (or says they've had enough), no matter how long it takes.

My partner asks, "Did you?" way too often. Just keep going and don't worry. I'll tell you when I'm done!

I've often been concerned about how long it takes me to reach orgasm, especially the first few times with a new partner. Once, after many unsuccessful attempts with a then-boyfriend, I expressed this concern. He reassured me that it doesn't matter how long it takes, that he can go for a very long time without getting tired. The next time we tried oral sex, having been relieved of that concern, I was able to have my first orgasm with him.

That said, you'll notice we recommend "a *reasonable* amount of patience." Some partners mistakenly interpret our advice as if the goal is an entry in *Guinness World Records* for Longest Licker. For your own sake and your partner's, be willing to change positions and make adjustments (add pillows, etc.) so you don't end up stiff and grumpy. Also, remember that not all people with a vulva can have orgasms, and not all can come from oral. If you give the impression that you're going to keep at it until the cows come home, your partner may feel forced to figure out a way to wrap things up.

If the guy is down there for a long time, I can never figure out if he wants to come up for air or if he's enjoying himself, so I usually end up faking an orgasm.

Okay, so some vulva-owners would be happy if you stayed there all night, and others get antsy far sooner. How can you tell the difference? Ask. If you're having trouble reading your partner's cues about whether they're enjoying every minute of it and just need more time or are ready to move on to something else, you can always whisper sweetly, "Would you like me to keep going? I'd be happy to, if you want."

Going Down: Dos and Don'ts for Partners

IF YOU FANCY dining downtown, don't take the express train straight from kissing to clit-licking. Work your way there gradually. Caress your partner's breasts or chest and spend some time licking or sucking their nipples. Kiss your partner's abdomen, belly, thighs, the crease where thigh becomes vulva. If your partner is wearing pants or underwear, breathing on the crotch or licking the fabric can be sexy. Once you're skin to skin, spend some time licking and kissing the outside of the vulva. Not only are you building anticipation and arousal, but you're also letting your partner know that you like their body, not just their "hot spots."

You're aiming for the clit eventually, but even when you have a thigh on either side of your head, don't jump directly to it. Explore the vulva with your mouth and tongue. Use your hands to gently open the outer lips if you need to. Lick all around slowly and appreciatively, as if the genitals were a delicious treat that you wanted to savor all over.

Once you've gotten that far, here are dos and don'ts from our survey's vulva-owners:

○ **DO focus on the external part of the clitoris, directly or indirectly.** The number one piece of advice was "Concentrate on the clitoris," "Lick the clitoris plenty," and "Stick to the outside: the clit!" In the space for oral sex advice, one respondent wrote simply, "Clit. Clit. Clit. Clit. Clit." Many more wrote variations of this:

> *I've had men try to use their tongue like they would their penis. Big mistake! The beauty of oral sex is that penetration isn't the only option. In fact, the main objective is clit stimulation.*

If you're not quite sure where to find the magic button, see page 61. Anatomy varies quite a bit from one person to the next, making some clits easier to find than others. If you're not positive, ask! You don't have to say, "Uh, honey? Where's your clitoris?" Rather, try saying, "Show me where it feels good to you," or asking, "Is this the place where it feels best for you?" Remember that the very tip of the clit is often too sensitive—your partner will likely prefer your attention to the shaft of the clitoris, or just off to one side or the other.

○ **DON'T get obsessed with the clitoris, though.** People with a vulva have somewhat conflicting preferences on this, but most say they want some attention to other parts of their vulva, not only their clit. Ask to be sure; after you've been going at it for a while, you can say, "Do you like it better if I just focus on your clit, or if I mix it up more?"

> *Act like you're French kissing my clit and labia. Suck on my labia. If I'm acting like I'm into it, don't change what you're doing, just keep right on at it.*

> *Caressing or kneading the thighs and getting the fingers involved are good ideas.*

> *Varying strokes and tempo is important. Touching around the clitoris is just as stimulating as actually touching it, if not more so.*

○ **DO be gentle, particularly at first.** Some partners make the mistake of diving directly for the clit and then licking ferociously. Instead of jumping in hard or fast, start out tenderly, licking gently. If you're not sure, ask, "Harder? Softer?"

I love when my partner acts like he's really into it and loves my pussy. That makes me feel sexy and more likely to come. And I cannot stress a gentle touch at first enough. A stronger touch should come only when the clit gets hard.

Don't push too hard on my clit. That thing is sensitive. A little goes a long way!

○ **DO incorporate your entire mouth.** This is another one of those subjects where taking your cues from porn is a mistake. In porn, the camera zooms in for a close-up of the performer sticking out their tongue and flicking the clit. This is for the pleasure of the porn viewer, not necessarily the person receiving the oral attention. In real life, people with a vulva say that lips, mouths, and the *flat* part of the tongue (not just the tip) can provide great stimulation too. In great oral sex in the real world (not for the cameras), the partner's face and mouth are usually too close to the vulva for an observer to see the tongue movements.

○ **DO let your fingers do the walking.** Most people with a vulva say they love the extra stimulation that fingers and hands can provide during oral sex. Depending on your position while your mouth is on your partner's vulva, you may be able to use your hands to stroke or massage their thighs, caress their breasts and nipples, or insert a finger or two in the vagina for G-spot stimulation, particularly once they're turned on.

I don't normally get an orgasm from just oral sex. It has to be combined with fingering.

Fingers are nice sometimes, but sometimes they're also distracting, especially when you're trying really hard to focus.

Stuff to Try

- Add zing to your lips, and your partner's nether ones, by chewing on Altoids, sucking on an ice cube, or sipping a warm liquid before going down. Fizzy liquids like sparkling water or sparkling wine can be a treat too.

  Sometimes when my partner is going down on me and I'm feeling stuck—like I'm not making progress toward coming—he'll take a drink from a glass of ice water and suck on some ice cubes for a minute or two. Then, when he goes back to licking my clit, his tongue feels really cool on my clit, which feels really good and sometimes is exactly what I need to get unstuck.

- Make dining down under even tastier by adding whipped cream, strawberries, kiwi, or anything else you can think of. Foods with oil in them aren't compatible with latex, but they're fine with plastic wrap. Although foods with high sugar content (like all the ones we just listed!) can increase the chance of a yeast infection, many people with a vulva tolerate occasional food play just fine. If your partner is particularly prone to yeast infections, play with food on their thighs and on the outside of their labia.

- Try humming over the clitoris—the vibrations can feel great. (But we bet you can't do it for long without laughing.)

○ **DO experiment with a variety of tongue motions to figure out what your partner likes best.** If they give it no thought, many partners settle into a methodical up-down lick, lick, lick routine disturbingly similar to a cat grooming itself. This may do the trick for some, but many prefer a bit of variety, especially early on. Try fluttering, flicking, slow steady strokes, circles and swirls, and listen for responses. You can also add variety to simple strokes by speeding up and slowing down, and changing the amount of pressure. If you find a stroke or two your partner likes a lot, stick with those. If your partner is being too quiet to give you feedback clues, easy-to-use check-in questions are "How's this?" and "Does this work?"

○ **DON'T go wandering once your partner lets you know you've hit the groove.** Many respondents had strong feelings about this, perhaps from being left in the lurch a few too many times:

> *DON'T STOP! The worst is when I'm almost "there" and the other person stops licking or moves to a different spot. I completely lose it and have to start over again. If I ask you not to stop or not to move ("Right there!"), then please don't unless you really need to come up for air. Don't just decide you're going to do something else for a while.*

> *Whenever a girl starts moaning or making noise (as long as it's pleasant noise), keep doing what you are doing. So many times, partners try something different when I start making noise and it just ruins the whole thing.*

○ **DON'T suck hard or bite.** Vulva-owners repeatedly say "Ouch!" to these techniques. While some people like gentle, brief sucking, many find it unpleasant. And save nibbling with your teeth for some other erogenous zone. Unless, of course, your partner asks you to bring on the biting.

> *Sucking is painful and should not be done. I think some men see it in pornography and assume that it feels good. It may to some, but it must be done VERY softly if at all.*

> *As much as guys don't want girls using teeth, girls don't want that either! It hurts.*

○ **DON'T rush or give up too soon.** You may have a mightily disappointed partner if you treat oral sex as a forty-yard dash to orgasm or a chore to be completed as quickly as possible to get ready for the ol' in-out. Instead, find a position that's going to be comfortable for you (see our earlier suggestions), and then take your time.

Should I Lick the Alphabet?

THE LICKING-THE-ALPHABET CUNNILIN-GUS technique was popularized by a comedian, Sam Kinison, but it's no joke. Licking each letter of the alphabet keeps the licker awake (a fact that should please any lickee) and hits lots of possible tongue angles and directions. It's probably best used as an information-gathering tool, rather than a surefire orgasm technique, because most people with a vulva want their partner to settle into a more consistent, repetitive motion when they're close to coming. One woman put it best when she told us on our survey, "The 'Oral Alphabet' is a good start. When your partner draws each letter on your genitals, focus on which letters feel the best and ask them to use those movements more frequently." Your partner might love a W motion, but don't be disappointed if you learn that a boring, repetitive set of I, I, I, I, I or a long string of hyphens is what really gets them hot.

I think people assume that everything has to be so fast to be erotic. It really doesn't. Going slow and gently massaging the genital area with your tongue is very erotic.

○ **DO connect after your partner comes.** If you've been down below for a while, it can be nice to cuddle and have some full-body contact after an orgasm. Some oral sex recipients like to taste their own juices in your kisses, but others don't, so check in about this. If you know your partner is in the latter category, wipe your mouth off on a tissue or the sheets, or have a sip of water before you snuggle up. Let your partner bask in orgasmic aftershocks and catch their breath before making it obvious that you're eager for them to return the favor. After a short pause, some people with a vagina love penetration after an oral sex-induced orgasm; others don't.

You with Your Head Between Those Thighs: You're (No Longer) Under Arrest

UNTIL 2003, ORAL sex was illegal in ten US states (Alabama, Florida, Idaho, Louisiana, Michigan, Mississippi, North Carolina, South Carolina, Utah, and Virginia). In four more states (Kansas, Missouri, Oklahoma, and Texas), different-sex couples were free to give each other as much oral as they pleased, but the identical act was illegal for same-sex couples. A now-famous Supreme Court decision, *Lawrence v. Texas*, declared all such laws unconstitutional, concluding that what consenting adults do in the privacy of their own homes is their own business. So, lick away, and breathe easy!

5

Going Deeper
Vaginal Penetration and Orgasm

Most people think penetration is how orgasms happen. And for most people with a penis, that's true: orgasms are pretty easy to come by (pun intended). The reality for people with a vagina, though, is starkly different: at least 70 percent of vagina-owners can't reliably orgasm from intercourse or any type of penetration alone.

That statistic leaves a lot of people wondering, "Why? Why is intercourse so *good* at providing orgasms for a penis, but so *bad* at providing orgasms for a vagina?" Or, as a lot of our audience members put the question to us, "Why don't I come during sex??!?"

The short answer is that penetration doesn't directly stimulate the most sensitive part of the clitoris, which is the part of the body most likely to lead to orgasm for people with a clit. The long answer—and what you can do about it—is the focus of this chapter.

Statistically speaking, vaginal intercourse is the most common partnered sexual activity. Of people over age eighteen in the United States, 89 percent have had it at least once in their lives, 64 percent have done so in the past year, and 52 percent boinked in the last month. Of course, there are plenty of people who aren't interested. Cis gay men, for example, have very low rates of vaginal intercourse for all the reasons you might guess—although some gay men are partnered with trans men who have a vagina, so penetration may (or may not) be part of their experience. Likewise, for most lesbians, penetration isn't a core focus of their sexual experience, but there are certainly plenty who enjoy penetration with fingers or a sex toy, or have a partner who happens to have a penis.

This chapter will focus on the largest demographic of people looking for help: people with a vagina who are looking to make intercourse with a penis more pleasurable, and more orgasmic, than it currently is. Much of it, though not all, is also relevant to a sex toy like a dildo or strap-on going inside a vagina. (There's more on using a strap-on on page 235.) If this combination of body parts and this activity is one that's of interest to you, read on! We realize it's not for everyone, so if this isn't a kind of sex that works for your body or appeals to you, then skip this chapter! We see penetration as only one option among many on the magnificent sexuality buffet.

Since people's experience with intercourse varies tremendously (as with all sexual matters), in this chapter you'll find:

○ Intercourse tips and positions that score extra points for clitoral pleasure
○ Lots of ideas for the majority of vagina-owners who find orgasms during intercourse tough or impossible to come by, strategies to tip the odds in your favor, and what to do if it just ain't happening
○ Tips for penis-owners on what people with a vagina want during intercourse
○ Advice for first timers

Positions for Penetration

WHAT'S THE BEST position for penetration? We hate to be the ones to break the news, but really, there's no such thing as a single best position. Why? Well, for one thing, the size, height, and lengths of the various body parts of the people involved make one couple's favorite position physically impossible for another couple. For instance, if a tall person with a penis and a short person with a vagina try to have doggie-style sex without finding a way to compensate for the height difference, the penis-owner may be thrusting into the air several inches above the vagina-owner's backside—not very satisfying for either of them. If the same couple turns their doggie-style position on its side, so they're both lying on their sides in spooning position, it can work great (more on that follows). So, the best positions for you and your partner tend to be ones where your bodies fit together in ways that feel great to *you*, which may be very different than for the couple next door.

Also, what feels good sexually varies dramatically from person to person. One vagina-owner may love the sensation of a partner's penis hitting up against the cervix (that's the deepest part inside the vagina). Another finds the sensation of having pressure against the cervix downright creepy. One person with a vagina may love how being on top lets them control the depth and angle of penetration, while another feels shy about being on top, as if they're all alone up there, blowing in the wind. Sex positions are like ice cream flavors: you get to choose your favorites, and as you travel through life, it's likely you'll discover new ones that are surprisingly good (yes, even if you're married or in a long-term relationship).

Most Popular Intercourse Positions

IN THIS CHART (page 145) and elsewhere in this chapter, we use the term *giver* to mean the person with the penis or strap-on who is doing the penetrating, and *receiver* to mean the person with the vagina who is being penetrated. The language people prefer for these roles constantly evolves. If these words aren't ones that seem right to you or aren't preferred as you read this, please substitute different ones.

NAME OF POSITION	HOW YOU DO IT	POPULAR MODIFICATIONS & TIPS
Missionary	Receiver lies on back, giver lies on top of them, chest to chest.	Legs up: Receiver rests legs against giver's chest or shoulders. Adding a pillow or two under the receiver's hips changes the angle, can also make the position work better for larger-bodied people.
Receiver on Top ("Cowgirl")	Giver lies on back, receiver straddles them and "sits on" penis/strap-on, facing giver.	Reverse cowgirl: Same position, but receiver faces giver's feet. Sometimes easier for larger people since no bumping of bellies. Receiver can lean forward or backward. Giver with a larger tummy can use a pillow under hips.
Doggie Style	Receiver kneels on hands (or forearms) and knees. Giver kneels or stands behind receiver, entering from behind.	Receiver lies flat on stomach, giver lies on receiver's back, supports self with arms, enters from behind. Can add pillows under hips. Experimenting with receiver up or lying flat, giver standing or kneeling, and using pillows under hips can also help modify this position for larger bodies and those with knee or back pain, arthritis, etc. Receiver can also rest chest on a large pillow or stool with pillows on it.
Sitting on Lap	Giver sits on bed or chair. Receiver straddles or sits on giver's lap, sitting on penis/strap-on.	Receiver can face toward or away from giver. Can be a great choice when receiver's body is heavier than giver's. Chair on a rug will slide less than on a slicker surface. A table or another chair nearby can be useful to hold onto.

What's Your Favorite Position for Intercourse?

WE ASKED OUR survey respondents what their favorite positions were for intercourse, and here's what they told us:

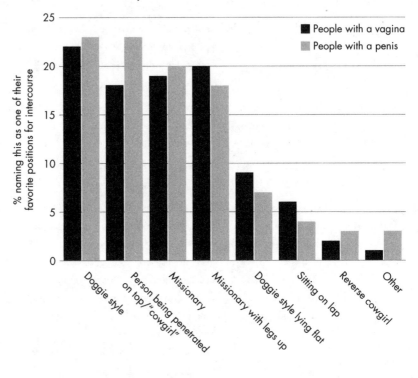

We were surprised by the nearly identical results, regardless of whether one is being penetrated or doing the penetration. The one exception is penis-owners showing a slight preference for their partner climbing on top.

Here's what people with a vagina told us:

I like that the missionary position allows me and my partner to be extremely close, and that we can hold each other and kiss while having sex. It also feels the best for me because positions that allow for deeper penetration often aren't comfortable for me.

I like sex on all fours from behind, with my head down. It allows for deep penetration. My partner can manually stimulate me, or I can do it myself, or he can play with my breasts. It's much easier to hit my G-spot in this position.

I actually really like being on the bottom, in missionary position. I like the security of having someone on top of me. I love being able to look up into someone's eyes and to be able to whisper into their ear that I love them or that I'm really enjoying what's happening. I like caressing their back and being able to watch what's going on down below. I also like being able to be a little rough from the bottom, either by scratching their back or by having them sort of elevate themselves above me and allowing me to thrust up to them. It can be very erotic and romantic all at once. And I love the collapse after the person on top has ejaculated. Feeling that weight on top of me just sort of completes it for me.

It depends on my mood. Sometimes I like him on top because I like to feel his weight on me; it's usually very intimate. Sometimes I like to take control and be on top. I get a better view of him, he can stimulate my genitals at the same time, I control the rhythm and the pace, and I can watch him orgasm. From behind is the best angle for the G-spot.

I love girl on top. I feel empowered. I can move the way I want to and set my own pace. Plus, both of his hands are free to touch me.

We asked people with a penis the same question about their favorite position for intercourse:

I like doggie style because I find it easier to touch my partner's sensitive spots while maintaining control. It's visually pleasing. I tend to last longer.

Missionary feels the most satisfying, and I enjoy seeing my partner's face when she's being pleasured. I enjoy kissing, sucking, and biting on her lips and neck while in that position.

Cowgirl is my favorite. It gives a nice view and many of my partners enjoyed it. I like when they lean forward to give a better angle of entry, and it usually feels good to both parties.

I can't think of what would be my favorite. I would say any position that includes face to face, because it allows me to feel more connected.

Other Positions to Try

IF YOU AND your partner haven't tested these already, here are four lesser-used positions definitely worth giving a whirl.

1. Crisscross. The receiver lies flat on their back with their knees bent. The giver lies sideways, with the receiver's bent knees over the giver's buttocks area (try having one of the receiver's legs just below the giver's butt, one leg just above). You can experiment with moving your heads closer together or farther apart to find the angle that feels best for you. Viewed from above, your bodies form a "T" or an "X" with your genitals joining where the lines cross.

Many couples love this position because it's relaxing—no one has to be "on top." It's easy for either partner to reach the clit. And the giver can easily control the depth and speed of penetration. It's also a perfect position for many who have joint pain—it's easy to add more pillows for support as needed—and works well for larger body sizes.

2. Tabletop or edge of bed. Find a table or another flat surface that's about as high as the giver's waist when standing up. Depending on height, the edge of the bed will work for some couples. The receiver lies on their back on the table or bed. You can use folded blankets on the table to add some padding, or use pillows under their head and/or butt to make it more comfortable or to adjust the crotch height. The receiver slides their butt to the edge of the table or bed, making it easy for the giver to insert from a standing position. Many receivers find this angle really comfortable because of the direct angle of penetration—there's less pulling and tugging on the skin around their vagina. It's also a good match for partners of size whose tummies sometimes get in the way, with the intimacy and connection of a face-to-face position.

What to do with the receiver's legs, other than let them dangle uncomfortably off the table? The more acrobatic among you may like to rest your feet on your partner's shoulders ("butterfly" position), or have your feet press against the giver's chest. A less physically demanding solution is to pull up two chairs and rest the receiver's feet on the chair backs or seats. Looking up or down at your partner in this position can be a real turn-on, and either partner has easy access to the receiver's clitoris.

Interestingly, sex swings, or slings, are designed specifically for the purpose of making it easy to get into this kind of position. Like a seated hammock, it hangs from the ceiling or attaches to a doorframe or a stand, suspended by ropes or chains. The receiver sits back in it, and the giver stands between the receiver's legs. Most swings include straps to support the receiver's legs and feet, and the swinging motion adds another dimension to penetration. If imagining the expressions on the faces of your landlord or visiting relatives doesn't inspire you to install a sex swing in your bedroom, a table is a camouflaged, multipurpose alternative.

3. Coital alignment technique (CAT). There's some evidence that this modified missionary position helps some people with a vagina have "Look, Ma, no hands!" orgasms. To use the technique, the giver is on top. Once inside, the giver "rides high" by moving their whole body up (toward the headboard) and to one side a bit. The giver lays their head and shoulders down flat rather than holding themselves up on their forearms. In this position, the base of the penis rubs against their partner's clitoris as the couple moves together. The couple finds a motion where they can rock together, the receiver rocking upward followed by the giver rocking downward, with the primary motion being the contact between the clit and the base of the penis. The giver's penis doesn't go as deep as with "traditional" intercourse thrusting—the movement is more up-and-down rather than in-and-out. Some couples find they can make it work with a combination of practice and luck.

If the man's body is positioned in a certain way during intercourse, it pushes up against an area of my body that allows me to orgasm.

I like it the best if my partner doesn't worry so much about hard thrusting. It's better if he focuses more on grinding his pubic bone against mine—it's a great source of clitoral stimulation!

Pillows Are Your Friend

PILLOWS ARE A valuable tool for anyone and can be even more valuable for people with a wide variety of issues involving pain, limited joint mobility, arthritis, or disabilities. You can use one or several pillows to support sore joints. Fat-positive advocates also recommend pillows for plus-size sex, to cushion knees, provide back support, raise a partner's hips or butt, and let gravity do the work of making genitals easier to access. A search for "sex furniture" and "sex pillows" will reveal a world of wedges, bolsters, and other shapes, as well as cushioned furniture designed to support bodies during sex. You can tie regular pillows or rolled-up towels with cord to create bolster shapes too.

4. Spooning. The spooning position is when your bodies fit together like two spoons in a drawer. (It's also a lovely way to cuddle, apart from intercourse.) Both people lie on their sides, facing the same direction, with the receiver in front, and the giver entering from behind. Some people call this position "doggie style on the side" because indeed, it has many of the advantages of traditional doggie style (easy to add clitoral stimulation, thrusting that gives G-spot stimulation, etc.) with some bonuses. It can work better than doggie style for couples with a big height difference, can be a great option for larger-sized bodies and those coping with pain or arthritis, and it's also less energy consuming for couples who want slower, more relaxed sex.

Spooning sex is great—it's so close, expressive, tender. Plus it's possible to do manual stimulation.

Beginner's Error

DON'T MAKE THE beginner's mistake of assuming that the more acrobatic the sex position, the faster the orgasms will fly. In fact, the reverse is often true, especially for people with a vagina: positions where you feel comfortable and relaxed are most likely to result in orgasms.

I like all the positions I've tried, except for ones that are so complicated to get into that you lose focus and arousal by the time you've gotten into position.

If you find it challenging to have orgasms during intercourse, simpler positions are nearly always better. Try an "is this really physically possible?" outrageous position on a day when you're in the mood to laugh or spice things up, but don't expect it to lift you to new orgasmic heights.

Invent Your Own Sex Position!

WHY LET THE people who write those "69 Hot New Sex Positions" web articles have all the fun? (Admit it: You've found yourself wondering what it must be like to get paid to brainstorm acrobatic sex positions, then give them outlandish names like "The Dangling Monkey" or "The Upside-Down Kumquat.") Here's how to play:

Start with a basic sex recipe:

○ Missionary
○ Cowgirl
○ Reverse cowgirl
○ Doggie style

- ○ Crisscross
- ○ Tabletop
- ○ Standing up
- ○ Sitting on lap
- ○ Parallel handstands

Add a twist:

- ○ Move your bodies closer together or farther apart (this generally changes the angle and depth of penetration).
- ○ Move one person up a little or down a little.
- ○ Move your legs closer together, farther apart, or over one partner's shoulders; wrap them around one person's body, or intertwine them.
- ○ Turn one of you in the other direction (like the difference between cowgirl and reverse cowgirl).
- ○ Lay the entire position on its side.
- ○ Try lying flat or boosting one or both of you up off the bed.

Consider a prop:

- ○ A chair
- ○ The edge of the bed
- ○ A bunch of pillows
- ○ The headboard
- ○ A tub or shower
- ○ The kitchen counter
- ○ Some other piece of furniture you own

Name it:

- ○ Almost as much fun as the position itself! Celebrities, tools, occupations, playground equipment, utensils, and furniture are all popular sources of inspiration.

We asked our survey takers who had a vagina and had had intercourse whether they had orgasms during intercourse, and if so, how they happened most often. Here's the breakdown of responses:

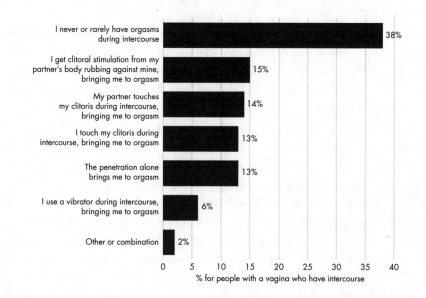

% for people with a vagina who have intercourse

What to Do About an Elusive Intercourse O

A LUCKY 13 percent of our survey respondents have an orgasm through penetration alone, without needing clitoral stimulation.

For me, the most incredible orgasms I've ever had have been from intercourse alone. I was surprised that the first time I had a really strong orgasm was my first time having intercourse!

I LOVE penetration! And I'm also a lesbian. A lot of my partners are surprised at first to find out it's my primary way of orgasming, but I'm like, the more the better, bring out the harness.

Although the Orgasms from Penetration Alone Club is statistically small, the desire to join it can seem like the top goal for many straight cisgender folks. Because the Club is the main experience you see in movies and porn, those excluded from it are often convinced they must be missing out.

Before we get any further, let us say it loudly and clearly:

It's *normal* for people with a vagina NOT to have orgasms from penetration alone. There is nothing wrong with you. Chances are most of your vagina-owning friends are having the same experience. You can have a fabulous, pleasure-filled sex life, a happy relationship or marriage, and lots of orgasms, without ever needing to have an orgasm from penetration.

But despite all that, maybe you still want to try. Even if it's not super common to have orgasms from penetration *alone*, 62 percent of our survey respondents said they were able to have orgasms *during* penetration at least some of the time. Here are our top tips for boosting the odds for people with a vagina:

1. Take control of your own orgasms. Maybe you were raised to believe that orgasms and sexual pleasure were things you'd begin to experience once you were married or in a serious relationship. Once you reached that life stage, you might have expected (consciously or not) that it's your partner's job to give you orgasms.

Of course, a great partner can absolutely help you have fantastic orgasms and boatloads of sexual pleasure. But it's easy to make the mistake of thinking that your orgasm is your partner's responsibility—that you can just lie back and enjoy. If you've internalized these ideas, you might blame your partner if you don't have orgasms. You might blame your partner if you have weak, inconsistent orgasms. And if you don't have a partner, well, you might figure you're just out of luck in the orgasm department.

We can't tell you how many people with a vagina have shared with us that the time their sex life blasted to a new level was when they started taking responsibility for their own orgasms. This is one area where vagina-owners could stand to learn a thing or two from cisgender, heterosexual men. In general, those men don't lie back, waiting hopefully for their partners to give them an orgasm—they rub or thrust in just the way they like, at just the right speed for them, at just the right rhythm, at their favorite angle. They initiate, negotiate, ask, or set things up so they can have sex in their favorite positions, the ones that give them their favorite kind of physical or visual stimulation. They think the thoughts and fantasize the fantasies that turn them on while they're having intercourse. They make it clear that they expect to have lots of sexual pleasure, and an orgasm, and they assume the sexual interlude will continue until they do. And if they don't have a partner, they take care of their own orgasm themselves.

If you have a vagina, changing the way you think about this stuff is *huge*. When you take charge of your orgasm, it means *you* take responsibility for making sure you get the kind of stimulation you need to have an orgasm while you're with a partner. You move your body in your favorite ways, think the thoughts, and fantasize the fantasies that will help you come. Some people with a vagina figure all this out when they're teenagers. Some figure it out when they're in their thirties. Some have to get married three times before they figure it out. But if you ask most confident, sexy, orgasmic vagina-owners what they do to have such satisfying sex lives, they'll tell you they stopped relying on the handsome prince, princess, or nonbinary royalty to have the pleasure map, and found the confidence to chart their own course.

2. Have your orgasm before or after intercourse. Many couples solve the problem of a person with a vagina not having orgasms through intercourse by spending plenty of time doing things focused on clitoral pleasure before or after intercourse. Performing oral sex before intercourse is particularly popular—there's even an

"Penetration" Without Penetration

FOR SOME PEOPLE, the energy of a certain act is more exciting than the need for the expected type of stimulation. This might include penetrating something that's not typically considered penetrable, or humping without penetration at all. For example, trans women who haven't had bottom surgery might want to experience being "fucked"—the sexual energy that word implies—without having to do so anally. Instead, they might lube their inner thighs and give their partner another option, which can still feel great for both parties.

entire book on the subject with the memorable title *She Comes First*. That way, you're highly aroused, and likely nice and wet, before penetration begins. Most people with a vagina find it perfectly comfortable, or even quite pleasurable, to have intercourse after they've already had an orgasm—they may even be able to come again now that they're warmed up.

You could also come by masturbating or using a vibrator during foreplay while your partner kisses and nibbles on your neck and shoulders, caresses your breasts and nipples, teases your mouth with a finger you can suck on, or adds other kinds of sensations you enjoy. If you haven't already come, your chances increase if you're highly aroused before intercourse begins. And if your partner comes first, that doesn't have to mean "game over"—together, you can continue to use fingers, hands, lips, tongues, and sex toys to let the fun continue if you want to come too.

3. Get the clit in on the action. This should be your number one take-home from our survey results on this subject: For people with a vagina who at least sometimes or always had orgasms during intercourse, 79 percent figured out a way to get clitoral stimulation while they went at it. This is your most powerful secret weapon to get over the orgasmic edge during penetration.

The easiest way for most to get that stimulation? Either you or your partner touch your clit with your fingers, hand, or a vibrator. Rather than feeling like this is a "second best" way to come, lots of couples recognize that it's not a big deal for the vagina-owner to need direct stimulation on this most sensitive area. Making a conscious effort to seek out intercourse positions that rub against the clit during penetration (or modify your angles so they will) can be a winning ticket.

Some people with a vagina tell us that part of the reason they settle for not coming during intercourse is because they're worried their partner would be offended if they reached down to polish the pearl while they're having sex. We needed to find out the truth. Do penis-owners really flip out if their partners reach down and add external finger action during penetration? We asked in our survey, and 80 percent of vulva-owners had given it a try.

Their experience was great: 98 percent who tried said they get either mostly or entirely a positive or an "I'm comfortable with that," no-big-deal, neutral type oZreaction from their partners. Many people with a vagina said their partners found it incredibly sexy to get to watch them pleasure themselves. So, wait:

A World of Sex Without Penis-Touching?

FOR THE VAGINA-OWNERS who can't orgasm from penetration alone, expecting them to have an orgasm *without* clitoral stimulation is like expecting a person with a penis to have an orgasm without any stimulation of their penis. Penises and clitorises develop from the same tissue as embryos. Anatomically, both are pleasure centers. Think of it this way:

Let's imagine an alternate universe that treats the penis as unimportant. In movies and porn, people in this universe watch penis-owners having explosive orgasms without penis stimulation. Instead, it's all about stimulation of their balls.

Let's say you're a penis-owner in this universe. You figure out how to masturbate when you're a teen, and you get pretty good at it, using the traditional penis-in-fist technique.

Then, you get a little older and have your first sex partner. The first time you hook up, your partner caresses your balls, licks your scrotum, focuses all their attention on that part of your body. It all feels great! You're super aroused. But it's not quite enough to reach orgasm. So, the interlude ends without an orgasm for you.

The same thing happens each time you and your partner get together. You keep trying new things to see whether they'll help you reach orgasm. You have extra-long sex sessions with your partner. You use fantasy. You squeeze and relax the muscles around your genitals. It's all really hot. But still no Os.

After a while your lack of orgasms leads you to start worrying that there's something wrong with you. Why isn't it working for you? You wonder if your partner would be offended if you reached down and rubbed your penis just a little while you were together. You have a hunch it might help. After all, you orgasm just fine when you masturbate.

> Seem absurd? It is. But this is the very real universe for many people with a vagina, most of whom grow up with the false "norm" that they should have orgasms from penetration alone. Expecting most or all people with a vagina to be orgasmic without clitoral stimulation (or without enough of the kind that works for that person's body) is as ridiculous as this alternative universe would be for penis-owners.

it's a turn-on for the penis-owner, and the clitoris-owner gets off? Talk about win-win sex!

During sex when I'm on top, touching my clitoris and building to an orgasm that way has been spectacular. My partner loved to watch me touch myself, especially when he could feel me clenching from inside. It also allowed us to time our climaxes together.

He's the one who wants me to! He loves to see me orgasm and knows that I know just what to do and he doesn't even need to worry about that part.

My boyfriend LOVES it. It really turns him on—if it's been going too long and I want him to finish, I touch myself and he's done in a minute or less!

But not all the news is so rosy. There were some who encountered partners who were threatened by vagina-owners taking matters into their own hands. Some people with a penis incorrectly think their partner self-touching is a sign of their own inadequate performance.

Some guys seem to be more open to it. Others think you just don't enjoy sex with them. If a guy doesn't like me to do it, it kind of makes me mad. I mean, I want to have an orgasm, too, dammit!

Most of the time, partners are okay with this, but my ex-husband was totally against it. He said if he couldn't make me orgasm without me touching myself, then why was he bothering? You notice, he's my EX-husband.

So, it's no wonder people with a vagina worry. Even if the vast majority of partners are supportive, they don't know whether theirs will be one of the small minority who will have a negative reaction. You want to let your fingers do the walking while you get it on together, but you're worried about how your partner will react? Here are some tips to get you started.

How to Start: Tips for the Clitorati

○ **Know your partner will probably be fine with it.** Boost your confidence by reminding yourself that most partners think it's hot. Here's what some penis-owners had to say:

> *It was pretty awesome. She came while I was having sex with her, which is an amazingly erotic experience.*

> *Before we tried it, I had never thought it would make me uncomfortable, but it did initially. I wondered, am I useless? But it was a lot of fun and she liked it a lot. I started to like it too.*

○ **Pick a good position.** The "traditional" missionary position with your partner's body lying flat on top of yours is often the worst for reaching your own clit—it probably doesn't give you space to move your hand the way you need to. Nearly any other position will work better: cowgirl, doggie style, crisscross, spooning, and so on.

Peeing After Vaginal Penetration: Useless Myth or Good Advice?

IT'S A COMMON question audience members ask us: "Should I pee after sex to prevent urinary tract infections (UTIs)?" The scientific evidence leans against, with research studies saying there's no proof it actually reduces the risk of a UTI. Nonetheless, the Centers for Disease Control (CDC) recommends it, and many vulva-owners swear by it based on their personal experience. Our conclusion: It can't hurt and might help, so go for it. But no need to interrupt a postcoital snuggle to rush to the john.

Also, if you know you can come via clitoral stim during masturbation, think about what positions tend to work well for you. Translating those into intercourse positions may improve your odds. For instance, if you've never masturbated in a kneeling position, practicing on your own so you'll know if it can work for you may be helpful before you try touching yourself in cowgirl position with your partner. Likewise, if lying on your front and rubbing against a pillow is your most effective technique on your own, try grinding in the same way while your partner enters you in a lying-down doggie-style position.

○ **Boost your partner's ego.** After your partner is inside you but before you touch yourself, load on the positive feedback. Use words and sounds to let your partner know how good it feels, how hot they look, and so on. (Don't fake or lie, of course—just be honest about what's good.) That reduces the chance your partner will feel threatened, because you're telling them that you're having a good time.

○ **Reach down with confidence.** Act like this is totally normal, just something people do. It is!

○ **Frame it as something fun and sexy.** If you feel like you need to say something as you first start touching yourself, try saying something like:

> "Are you one of the people who thinks it's hot if I touch myself while we_____ [fill in favorite slang for having sex]?"

> or

> "Let's see whether we can both come."

> or

> "I need a little extra help to be able to come—you feel *so good,* I really want to come with you."

It's unlikely your partner is going to say, "No, it doesn't turn me on to watch you touch yourself" or "No, I don't want you to come." If you say things like this, you're giving your partner a positive (and accurate) way to look at what's going on, which reduces the chance they'll get scared or insecure. Of course, it's also fine just to reach down without saying anything at all.

> *My boyfriend helps me while I masturbate by fingering me and he can be a part of it. We just tried having sex while I touched myself down there and for the first time we had simultaneous orgasms.*

○ **Invite your partner to help.** You can just put your partner's hand there and keep your hand over it to show how you like it. Or try saying, "Does it work for you to touch my clit at the same time?" Your partner will likely need a bit of direction about what feels good once you get their fingers in the right place. See the box Whose Fingers? (page 162) for more on this.

○ **Ask your partner to slow down, if needed.** Some people with a vagina find the sensation of constant thrusting distracting; they need to be able to concentrate on their clitoral sensations to get over the edge. If this is the case for you, you can ask your partner temporarily to slow their thrusts way down, or just stay still inside you, moving just enough to stay hard. Then, as your orgasm begins to swell up inside you, you can whisper sweetly, "I'm ready for you," or use one of those great porn lines like "Oh, fuck me, fuck me!" Chances are they'll be happy to oblige.

"But I Want to Come from Penetration Alone!"

AFTER A TYPICAL college speaking engagement, the audience files out, and a handful of people stay behind to talk with us. One question comes up without fail: "But I *really* want to come from penetration alone—no hands, no vibrator. Isn't there *something* I can do?"

If you haven't guessed by now, we think that if penetration doesn't lead you to O-land, you're best off enjoying penetration for itself and pursuing orgasms in other ways. But if you insist, here are techniques that some people with a vagina

Whose Fingers?

MANY COUPLES WHO combine clitoral stimulation with intercourse find it works well if the vagina-owner takes care of providing the stimulation because that's the partner who knows precisely what, where, and how to touch that feels just right. But lots of people with a vagina enjoy or even prefer having their partner's fingers on their clit during intercourse. What works best is a matter for each pair to figure out.

She can bring herself to orgasm much better than I can usually because she's the most familiar with her own body. Also, I tend to get distracted when doing multiple things at once, and if it's me rubbing the clitoris, then often I get distracted and stop, or at the very least, do it haphazardly.

I touch the woman's clitoris as much as she directs me to, which varies by partner. The easiest positions are generally ones where I enter her from behind and can reach around in front of her to stimulate her clit.

I've touched it, he's touched it. This ought to be a regular part of sex if I'm going to get off! If he's not invested in me getting off, I won't be having sex with him again. Who's doing it changes depending on the position. It's easier for me to touch it spooning style while it's easier for him to touch it girl-on-top style.

Of course, not all people with a vagina want or need clitoral stimulation during intercourse. Some respondents on our survey said they found it distracting. For some couples, the answer to "Whose fingers?" may simply be "Neither."

say have worked for them to learn how to come during penetration without the assistance of a hand or a sex toy:

○ **Get hot and bothered.** Some find it helps to be really, really turned on already, through oral sex, masturbation, or some other type of stimulation before intercourse begins (or even earlier in the day, before they see their partner). Starting the action at a higher level of arousal means there's less distance to travel to reach the finish line. For some, having an orgasm before intercourse makes it easier for them to come again during it.

○ **Try the coital alignment technique.** CAT, as it's known, has ardent fans who swear by it as the route to orgasm during intercourse. While it takes practice and doesn't work for everyone, it's definitely successful for some couples. See page 149 for more.

○ **Be creative.** Experiment with positions to find pleasurable ways your partner's body can grind against your clit. You might rub against your partner's pelvic bone or the shaft of the penis during intercourse, regardless of who's on top. You may find the angle of penetration makes a difference in terms of how much and what kind of clitoral contact you get.

I like being on top at a slight angle above him. I practically lie on him. I can really grind on him this way and our heads don't get in the way.

Girl on top didn't work for me to come until I tried dangling one leg off the bed. That gives me deeper penetration and more solid clit contact.

○ **Grind your pelvis.** Moving your body can also help; there's some evidence that pelvic motion may increase the chance of orgasm for at least some people with a vagina. At the very least, moving your pelvis may help you grind against your partner or increase clitoral contact—or just make your sex more energetic and enthusiastic!

○ **Teach your body.** You can try to teach yourself to associate the sensations of penetration with orgasm. Start by having intercourse with clitoral stimulation from your own hand. A second before you come, stop the clitoral stimulation, and allow your partner's thrusting to be the thing that pushes you over the edge to orgasm. If that works, the next time, you do the same thing, but stop the clitoral stimulation two seconds before you fall over the orgasmic edge, and let the thrusting carry you to orgasm. Over a period of weeks or months, you continue getting yourself highly aroused, most of the way to orgasm, but over time, rely on intercourse to take you more and more—and maybe eventually most or all—of the way there. You can also practice this using a dildo or other object for penetration.

○ **Legs together.** Experiment with closing your legs once your partner is inside. Changing leg positions, and possibly squeezing your leg muscles, can increase the sensation you get. Your partner can straddle your closed legs rather than your partner's legs being together inside your spread legs.

Location, Location, Location

THERE SEEMS TO be some evidence that the location of the clitoris—slightly higher or slightly lower on the body, and slightly closer or farther from the vagina—may affect one's ability to have an orgasm during intercourse. The clitoris-owner can't control this any more than any of us can control the distance between our eyes or length of our shins; it's just a matter of genetics and prenatal development. Researchers theorize that this may be one of many factors that make it easy for some people with a vagina to have orgasms from penetration, while others can't.

Clitoral size, on the other hand, does not seem to matter.

The best way for me to come during sex is in the missionary position with my legs crisscrossed.

○ **Try a ball.** Try putting a small, soft ball like a Hacky Sack on the clitoris as a way to add pressure during missionary position sex, increasing the contact between the top partner and the clit.

○ **Lose control.** One woman told us she was finally able to have orgasms during intercourse when she let go of the need to "control her own orgasm" and instead stayed intensely focused on the sensations she was feeling from her partner.

○ **Focus on yourself.** It helps some people with a vagina to stay focused on their own pleasure and not worry so much about pleasing their partner. It's okay not to be an award-winning lover every minute. In fact, it may free you up to stay in your own groove if you take a break from running your hands over your partner's body, or stop worrying about moving your body the way you know they like.

○ **Find the right rhythm.** Often, the pace of intercourse is controlled by the penetrating partner, but most people with a vagina need their own consistent, steady rhythm to be able to have an orgasm. Try positions where you can more easily control the rhythm (e.g., cowgirl or, for some, doggie style). You can give your partner feedback about what speed feels best to you, or grasp your partner's hips or butt to help control the motion.

○ **Use your mind.** The mind is a powerful thing in the quest for orgasms. Find the images or stories that turn you on, and use them while you're having sex with your partner. For more about the wonders of using your own imagination, see page 38.

One or two of these tips might work for you. Or none of them may work. Keep in mind that though coming hands-free during intercourse can be fun, there's no rule that says it's the best way. If you're the kind of person who has orgasms relatively easily, from a wide variety of kinds of stimulation, you're more likely to find these techniques may work for you. If, on the other hand, you're somebody whose body has more specific requirements—you need good, long stimulation of just the right spot with exactly the right motion and the perfect amount of lubrication—it'll probably be more difficult for you to replicate those conditions. And that's okay too.

The Myth of the Vaginal Orgasm

ONE HUNDRED YEARS ago, Sigmund Freud made a mistake when he declared the existence of the "vaginal orgasm" and wrote that it was far more desirable than its sorry cousin, the clitoral orgasm. Plenty of people throughout human history have been wrong about things: The early Greeks believed the world was flat. Orville and Wilbur Wright first built airplanes that didn't fly. In colonial times, many people slept propped up because they thought they'd die if they lay flat. Today, we see these other errors as quaintly misguided. But for some reason, the mistaken concept of the vaginal orgasm hasn't faded away.

It's now well established that there's only one kind of orgasm for people who have a vagina. Certainly, different kinds of stimulation can bring on an orgasm, and various different nerves can be involved. An orgasm with or without penetration, with or without a vibrator, with or without extended tantric breathing, can *feel* very different. But what's happening in your body once the waves of sensation begin is the same, no matter what kind of stimulation brought it on. The clitoris—including the clit's internal and external structures—is responsible for all orgasms, even those that happen during intercourse. And the muscles of the vagina are involved in most orgasms once the orgasm begins.

The Wonders of Lube

LUBE IS ONE of those secrets to great sex that many people wish they'd discovered much earlier in their lives. Lubricant makes things slide better—and therefore feel better—by reducing friction during sex. Vaginas have the ability to lubricate all by themselves, which can be a very lovely thing.

But things slide better against each other if *both* surfaces are wet rather than a wet surface sliding against a dry surface. Using lube isn't a sign that something is amiss, any more than shaving with shaving cream is a sign of weakness.

It's also important to realize that vaginas vary widely in the amount of wetness they produce. Some get really wet really quickly; for others, it's much slower or hardly at all. It may vary based on the phase of your menstrual cycle, stress, drugs, alcohol, age, menopausal status, or nothing at all. It's a normal process of aging that vaginas don't tend to get as wet as they used to. No shame, just life! And on top of all that, wetness doesn't tell nearly as much as you might guess about how turned on the vagina-owner is—for more about that, see page 31.

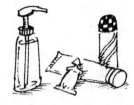

Adding lube to a vagina, vulva, and/or penis is exactly what you need for penis-in-vagina sex when the vagina isn't extremely wet. Lube can also help if you're having a longer sex session, having rougher sex, when you're using condoms or sex toys (which can dry things out a little), or anytime you just want to make sure penetration stays nice and slippery—which for most people is just about every time!

We're not talking about the lube that comes on a lubricated condom, though that's a start—we mean lube you buy in a bottle or tube near the condoms in a pharmacy or supermarket, purchase from a sex toy store, or order online. Some particularly lube-friendly sex stores (such as those listed on pages 215–216) have lube sampling stations with lots of lube brands where you can put a few drops on your fingertips and rub it around for a while to see which consistency, scent, and skin feel you like best.

Lube is great for penis-in-vagina sex, essential for anal sex, and an excellent option for playing with sex toys. Lots of people with a vagina use lube (or their own saliva) for masturbation too. For intercourse, you use lube by putting it on the penis (on top of the condom or directly on the penis if not wearing a condom) and/or around the entrance to and inside the vagina. Adding a drop of lube inside a condom can add sensitivity for the person wearing the condom. Putting lube on the clit underneath a dental dam or plastic wrap can also feel good. Because doing so decreases friction, it reduces the chance that a condom will break, so adding lube when you're using condoms actually makes sex safer.

The very first time you have intercourse is a fantastic time to use lube because it makes everything slide better and can make the first time more comfortable. Too bad most people having sex for the first time don't even know lube exists! And at a different stage of life's journey, vaginal tissue may get thinner with age, making it more susceptible to tearing. Lube helps reduce that risk too.

There are three basic kinds of sexual lubricants: water-based, oil-based, and silicone. Water-based is the most popular for most situations. It's totally safe to use with latex condoms, and if it dries out a little while you're using it, you can just add some water to rejuvenate it (some couples keep a spray bottle next to the bed for a quick spritz). Some water-based lubes contain glycerin, a sugar, which some find can cause yeast infections. If you find yourself prone to yeast infections, you may want to seek out the glycerin-free kind. Glycerin is particularly common in flavored lubes, which are fun for oral sex but not as good for vaginal sex.

Most oil-based lubes are homemade inspirations: massage oil, coconut oil, hand lotion, chocolate sauce, and so on. There are also a small number of store-bought oil-based lubes, mostly advertising coconut oil. Oil-based lubes are fine for use on a penis for masturbation or oral sex, and for anal play if you're not using latex safer sex supplies. Coconut oil also has fans as an option for vulvas and vaginas.

Others raise concerns that coconut and other oils aren't a good match for vaginas because of a possible increased risk of yeast infections, since oil can trap bacteria. Oily lubes also aren't safe to use with latex condoms because oil breaks down latex, so your condom could break (that means no chocolate sauce cunnilingus followed by a romping session of condom-based intercourse).

Silicone lube is the newest addition to the lube party. It's safe with condoms, doesn't dry out as quickly as water-based lube, and can even be used underwater (ooh! ahh!). Some people find silicone lubes feel warmer because they transmit heat better. They cost more than water-based lubes, and you need soap and water to wash them off. If you want to use silicone lube with a silicone sex toy, some say to put a condom on it, claiming the silicone-silicone chemical reaction could melt your favorite toy. The risk of a silicone meltdown in your bedroom might be a bit overblown—the dildo that used to stand tall is not actually at high risk of melting into a puddle on the floor. If you have a silicone lube

A Sex Ed Party Trick

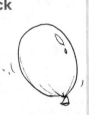

HERE'S SOMETHING TO amuse you and your friends when you're hanging out late at night. Blow up two nonlubricated latex condoms like balloons and tie them off. Onto one condom balloon, wipe some water-based lube. Onto the other, wipe something oil based (petroleum jelly, vegetable oil, hand lotion, etc.). Make sure you know which balloon is which.

Put them aside in a place where you can see them. Talk among yourselves. At some point later that night, the condom balloon with the oily lube will pop all by itself because oil breaks down the latex over time.

And that, friends, is why you should never use oil-based lube when you're using latex condoms!

If Penetration Hurts

WHEN A PERSON with a vagina tells us penetration is painful for them, we typically start exploring things like:

- Is there enough foreplay? Vaginas need to be aroused before penetration begins. They literally make more space as they get aroused, a process called "tenting."

- Is the penis or sex toy entering the vagina slowly? Some vaginas need to relax and adjust to having something inside.

- Are they adding plenty of lube?

- Is the painful penetration too fast and hard? Most receivers don't enjoy jackhammering.

In our experience, most problems related to pain during penetration can be solved with questions along these lines.

But in some cases, the cause is a medical issue like vaginismus or vulvodynia. Vaginismus is when the vagina tightens in an involuntary muscle spasm as penetration is attempted. For some people with a vagina, vaginismus is an issue they've grappled with even before trying to have penis-in-vagina sex: they also find inserting a tampon or finger painful or impossible.

While vaginismus is triggered by penetration, vulvodynia is chronic pain around the opening of the vagina. It's often described as a burning or stinging sensation. To be officially classified as vulvodynia, it can't be a onetime or occasional experience—the person would need to have symptoms for at least three months.

To be clear, both these diagnoses are more than feeling a little sore after sex, or having penetration hurt a bit. They're conditions that persist over months and years, and, in the case of vulvodynia, can make riding a bicycle or a horse, or even something as simple as wearing jeans uncomfortable or painful.

For trans masculine folks with vaginismus, dysphoria may be an underlying factor and can also make it more difficult to seek treatment, as these two respondents to our survey noted:

> I have vaginismus, so any vaginal penetration is extremely painful. I fully believe dysphoria makes it worse for me. It's an aspect of sexuality I haven't explored because it's so scary and I don't trust medical professionals to help me with it while respecting my identity.

> I have bottom dysphoria and vaginismus so severe that, between the neurological pain of being touched there and the vaginismus, they have to use the baby speculum on me at the GYN. I wasn't able to touch my genitalia for cleaning until I was nearly 15, and could only make cursory contact until I was 24. It's been incredibly freeing to embrace the idea I never need to receive penetration at any point in my life to have meaningful sex with other men. That, for the first time, lets me see my body as whole, not flawed and in need of fixing.

Too often, trans and nonbinary people put off seeking medical attention because of fears of misunderstanding, misgendering, and/or mistreatment. As conversations continue to evolve around inclusion and representation, many in the medical field are learning how to be more affirming and supportive of their trans and nonbinary patients. We suggest looking into local LGBTQ centers and/or resource groups to help find doctors who are competent in both the care you need and affirming practices.

If any of this resonates with you, no matter what your gender identity, we'd suggest reading more to see whether more detailed descriptions of these diagnoses seem to fit your experience. Finding effective treatments for pain can take time but is certainly worth the investment! For the best results, you should seek and integrate the advice of three types of specialists: a gynecologist who specializes in pain, a physical therapist experienced in pelvic-floor therapy, and a sex therapist. For a list of websites that can help you find these professionals, check this book's website.

you love, and a silicone toy you love, just test a little bit of lube on a (nonessential) corner and see what happens. It may be fine.

Most vagina-owners tell us they don't like warming gels and lubes (products that warm up with breath or rubbing). Many who've tried one say that instead of feeling gently warm, it was burning hot! Some brands are milder than others, though, and a few like the way they get their blood flowing. If you're curious, you may want to experiment with different kinds and start with a tiny dab to prevent a fiery surprise.

Simultaneous Orgasms

AH, SIMULTANEOUS ORGASMS. Like performing stand-up comedy or getting a baby to sleep through the night, coming at the same moment is easier said than done. Often the work involved requires the partner who tends to come faster going cross-eyed trying to hold back while the partner who tends to take longer tries every trick imaginable to speed up. In the end, if both people do succeed in coming simultaneously, they may just decide they were working so hard that they didn't get to have very much fun.

In ancient Greece, Hippocrates believed that simultaneous orgasms were necessary for conception, inventing the goal that many modern couples still aspire to. Now that we know that people with a uterus can get pregnant regardless of the timing or existence of their orgasms, there's no reason that coming at the same time is better than any other way. (Besides, most couples having intercourse these days aren't hoping to get pregnant.) Sure, simultaneous orgasms can be fun, but

Your Body Wants to Get You Pregnant

MANY PEOPLE WHO menstruate find they're horniest around the most fertile time of their cycle, the days before they ovulate. Why? A combination of high levels of estrogen and lots of slippery, wet cervical fluid (healthy vaginal secretions) combine to pump up your libido. It's nature's way of trying to seduce you into having sex—and getting you pregnant. (This effect may be different or nonexistent if you're on a hormonal form of birth control or hormone replacement therapy [HRT].)

Want to be able to tell with confidence when you're fertile and when you're not, even if your menstrual cycles are irregular? We recommend the book *Taking Charge of Your Fertility* by Toni Weschler—it rocks our socks. If you're having the kind of sex where a sperm could come into contact with an egg, but you don't want to get pregnant, check iloveorgasmsbook.com for great sources on exploring birth control options.

they're not evidence that two people were made for each other, trophies for award-winning sex, or markers of true love.

Many couples find they actually enjoy their orgasms more if they don't even try to make them happen at the same time. With the "sequential orgasm" approach, partners alternate their focus between one person's pleasure and the other. The one being pleasured gets to luxuriate in the sensations without worrying about either racing or holding back. The one helping to provide pleasure gets the fun of the sights and sounds of their partner getting really turned on and having an orgasm. If the orgasms just happen to coincide, these couples certainly enjoy them, but they let go of the simultaneous goal most of the time.

If you and your partner do decide to try to come together, the best strategy for couples having penis-in-vagina sex is usually to have the person with a penis handle the timing. It's much harder for a person with a vagina to control the speed and timing, but if you're a penis-owner with finely tuned ejaculatory control (for more on how this works, see page 311), you may be able to get yourself close to orgasm and then hover around that arousal level for a while until your partner cues that they're getting close. Once the vagina-owner's orgasm starts, the penis-owning partner can try to join in quickly.

What Is Tantric Sex?

TANTRIC SEX IS a sexuality practice that emphasizes spirituality and energy exchange between two people. Rooted in India and various Eastern religions, tantric sexuality belief systems, approaches, and techniques are diverse. They often include slow, ritualized breathing; extended eye contact between partners; and aspects of yoga, meditation, and focused self- and partner-awareness. It's possible to spend a lifetime studying tantra, and there are countless books, websites, and workshops where you can learn more if the subject interests you.

We began with intense foreplay that involved slowly touching each other's body for a really long time. After this, we were so in tune to each other's needs that the sex was slow and passionate. We breathed in unison, finished together. It was fantastic.

Some practitioners say tantric sex revolutionizes and enhances their sex life, shifting the focus away from seeing erection, ejaculation, and orgasm as goals, and instead allowing them to make love for far longer, feel a deeper and more intimate connection with their partner, and "channel the divine energy of the universe." Others say it's just not their thing, preferring the attitude of the book called *Life's Too Short for Tantric Sex.*

My partner gets me almost there with his fingers and with his penis inside me or almost inside me, so that he is ready to come when I do. We lie side by side. We don't do this all the time, but it's a really nice treat.

Degendering Penetration

FOR A LOT of people, penetrative sex comes with gender role expectations. (We're focusing on frontal penetration in this chapter; for more on anal check out Chapter 11.) Many have done work to unlearn such expectations and societal norms, but it can bring up mixed feelings for trans and nonbinary folks. In our survey, 30 percent of cis people with a vagina said their favorite way to have an orgasm was intercourse combined with clitoral stimulation. For trans folks with a vagina, that percentage dropped to 4. One trans masculine respondent to our survey summed it up this way:

Penetration might not exactly trigger dysphoria, but I know my brain doesn't see it as something masculine.

For others, the negative reaction was even stronger:

As a trans man, front hole penetration is an absolute no. In fact, it's difficult for my genitals, including my dick, to be touched directly in a way that isn't something I experience as a form of pain.

Vaginal penetration is a trigger; the idea gives me anxiety attacks sometimes.

But not everyone deals with dysphoria, and even those who do don't all experience it the same way. Some trans masculine people really enjoy frontal penetration and find it works for them.

My favorite way to have an orgasm is to have my girlfriend penetrate me while my clit is stimulated, preferably both anal and vaginal penetration.

Being out as trans and with other people who get trans people finally let me open up to have vaginal orgasms. I never liked penetration until I knew my partners didn't see my genitals as a defining characteristic of my gender. Now I'm all about penetration!

Sometimes the biggest challenge is other people's assumptions. Some partners might see a vagina and assume the owner wants it penetrated. Some partners might see a penis and assume the owner wants to use it for penetration. While that is the case for some trans and nonbinary people, it certainly isn't true for all—nor is it true for all cis people with these body parts!

I do not have bottom surgery, and lots of people assume that my genitalia works the same as a cis man's does, or that I'd want primarily penetration in a sexual relationship and assume I'm a top. I just explain that their assumptions are wrong, and that it can be harmful to make assumptions like that. Sex isn't all about penetration, and just 'cause someone has a penis doesn't mean that's what they want/enjoy.

With partners who are queer it's usually easier because they are more open to the idea that parts aren't prescriptive. But people still sometimes think that my identities mean a certain thing, or that having a vagina means I must like vaginal penetration. I talk to people and try not to fuck with anybody who can't wrap their head around all that.

Tips for Partners with a Penis

IF YOU HAVE a penis and your partner has a vagina, here are some tips for increasing your partner's pleasure and chances of reaching orgasm.

○ **Slow it down.** When we asked our survey takers with a vagina what advice they would give to a partner about how to make penetration more pleasurable, they overwhelmingly said things like "Don't rush!" and "It's not a race to the end." Many penis-owners get the mistaken impression from porn that people with a vagina want hard, fast pounding.

○ **Make foreplay last.** This was the second most common tip our respondents said they'd like to give penis-owners. If your partner isn't extremely aroused, it's too soon to start penetration. Because vaginas elongate as they get turned on, entering your partner before their body's ready can be uncomfortable or painful.

Foreplay is the absolute most important part of any kind of sex for me, especially intercourse.

Foreplay foreplay foreplay! Get the girl super excited so that she is BEGGING you to enter her. When it finally goes in, it feels AMAZING!

Many people with a penis have gotten the memo that foreplay is important, but don't spend enough time on it. They may perform oral sex for a few minutes, and then pop back up, with a proud look on their face, "See, I did it—oral sex! Foreplay!" Meanwhile, their vagina-owning partners are often thinking, "Uh, thanks, but that's not nearly enough time to build the arousal I need." Also, foreplay doesn't need to be something that just happens when the bedroom door is closed—it can build up all day, with flirting, teasing, sexts, and anticipation.

○ **Bring lube.** Ask your partner whether it's okay to put some on your penis. It may not make much difference for you, but lube often makes penetration far more comfortable for the person being penetrated.

○ **Ease in slowly, a bit at a time.** Many people with a vagina—even those who love intercourse and have had lots of it—complain that penis-owners push in too hard and too fast.

Be gentle. Give her time to adjust to you.

○ **Experiment.** Find out what speed, depth, rhythm, angle, and strength of penetration your partner likes. Try slow, sensuous thrusts; lots of in and out near the entrance of the vagina; or staying deep inside your partner while you move back and forth a shorter distance. If fast, hard thrusts are what you're used to from masturbation, you can "retrain" yourself by practicing masturbating with a slower, wetter, somewhat looser hand, more like the stimulation you'd get from a vagina.

○ **Ask for feedback.** Say to your partner, "Do you like it better when I move like this, or like this? Does this feel good?" Don't be silent because you think it's unromantic to talk—the third most common piece of advice people with a vagina said they'd like to tell their partners was to talk to them more! This doesn't mean they want an endless stream of chatter (they don't), but checking in now and then is appreciated.

> *I think communication is the sexiest part of intercourse. Talk to me and ask me what I want. Tell me how I make you feel. All of these things make it a lot sexier and also help to make sure we're both feeling okay and getting what we want from the experience.*

> *Tell me how to pleasure YOU. Chances are, I'll be more open about what feels good for me, too.*

○ **Stay tuned in during intercourse.** Kiss and caress your partner, whisper sweet things in their ear. Enjoy the emotional closeness and intimacy. Pay attention to your partner's sounds, movements, and other nonverbal clues about what they like and how they're doing.

> *Don't just fixate on my vagina and clitoris, but touch my breasts, my face, my neck—show me you care by being gentle and passionate.*

○ **Know that most people with a vagina don't come from intercourse alone** (we know, we're repeating ourselves!). Don't assume there's something wrong with you, and definitely don't imply there's something wrong with your partner!

○ **Realize longer isn't always better.** If you have some control over how long sex lasts, don't assume your partner wants you to keep thrusting all night long. Some people with a penis mistakenly think that if they can pump away for long enough, they're sure to generate an orgasm. But most people with a vagina say that if their partner lasted for twenty hours of intercourse, they still wouldn't have an orgasm because they're not getting the right stimulation. People who answered our survey were more likely to complain about "marathoners" who left them sore than ones who came too soon.

○ **Develop ejaculatory control.** On the other hand, if a partner with a vagina *is* able to have orgasms through intercourse, the longer you can last, the more likely it is that they'll have enough time for the sensations to build up to an O. So, if it usually takes a given partner with a vagina, say, seventeen minutes to have an orgasm, but you explode seventeen *seconds* after penetration begins, your partner is clearly a long way from being able to have an orgasm during intercourse. Most people with a penis find it helpful to have some degree of ejaculatory control, which is why we address this further on page 311. But just because it's handy to be able to choose when you will or won't come doesn't mean this is the critical factor that determines whether your partner will come or not.

Because vaginas can get sore and an orgasm might never happen when intercourse lasts *too* long, a penis-owner who's mastered ejaculatory control should check in from time to time: "Would it feel good if I kept going, or should I come now?"

○ **Be supportive of your partner getting clitoral stimulation during intercourse.** Just as penetration itself likely gives you the stimulation you need to come, clitoral stimulation is most likely what your partner needs. Experiment to see whether there are positions or angles that work better to get the clit in on the action. Encourage your partner to touch their clit while you're going at it, or massage it gently yourself with wet fingers. If your partner uses a vibrator to masturbate, welcome it into your bed together as a fun way to rev up your sex life and amplify your partner's pleasure. Unless your penis has its own vibrating feature, there's no reason to feel competitive with a toy.

We usually make sure one of us is touching her clit at all times. The best position for her to touch it is doggie style; the best for me is a modified missionary position where I sit upright and put more weight on my knees. This position is also good for hitting her G-spot.

○ **Find a brand, size, and style of condom you like.** Bring a couple with you. Take the initiative for putting it on rather than waiting to see whether your partner requests it. If you need to, get used to the sensations of coming with a condom on (and road test a bunch of different brands to find the one that fits you best) by wearing one to masturbate. You can get a bunch of different condoms by searching online for "condom variety pack" or "assorted condoms."

> *Learn to put on a condom in the dark. Girls don't really practice it, so guys need to be an expert at it.*

○ **Finally, don't assume that intercourse should happen every time (or even most times) you have sex.** Be open to having your orgasm other ways, like oral sex, rubbing against your partner's body, getting a hand job, or masturbating while you're together. People with a vagina tell us that when they're not in the mood for intercourse, they'd often be happy to bring their partner to orgasm some other way. But if they feel like intercourse is the only option, they'll opt out of sex altogether.

Intercourse During Pregnancy

IT'S PERFECTLY SAFE to have intercourse and orgasms any time while you're pregnant—right up until the water breaks before the baby's birth! (This assumes the pregnant person hasn't had problems with this or past pregnancies. If they have, discuss the topic of sex and pregnancy with your midwife or doctor.) During penetration, a penis or sex toy can't reach or touch the baby.

When a pregnant person is near or past their due date, intercourse that includes a partner ejaculating inside can be an effective way to encourage labor to begin. Semen contains prostaglandins, the same substance that doctors apply to the cervix to induce labor artificially. The same activity that got the baby in there can also help get the baby out!

Twelve Steps to Making Your First Time a Great Time

ARE YOU A person with a vagina thinking about having intercourse for the first time? Here are our top twelve tips for making the first time something you'll want to remember.

1. **Do it because you want to.** Not because your friends have already done it. Not because your partner wants to. Not because you think you're too old to be a virgin. It's normal to have mixed feelings—nervousness, excitement, fear, anticipation—but fundamentally, it should be because of your desire, not any external or internal pressure to do it.

   Make sure that this is the right time and the right person. Ask yourself, if this ends today will I regret having had sex with him?

   Don't rush into it just because you think you have to. I thought I was too old to be a virgin (twenty-one) and that there was something wrong with me. So the first chance I got, I went for it. Stupidly.

2. **Be with a partner you trust.** The people who have the most positive memories of their first intercourse experience say they did so with a partner with whom they shared mutual trust, respect, and caring. Having this kind of relationship sets the stage for the rest of our advice on this subject.

   I think we were both nervous because we were both virgins. It actually didn't hurt as bad as I thought it would. It was a little awkward because it was our first time, but it was still good because we really love each other and we were comfortable with each other.

Please, please only have sex for the first time with someone you're in a relationship with and love and feel immensely comfortable with. It's a somewhat physically uncomfortable experience, so that won't be satisfying, but the emotional experience will be.

Choosing to lose my virginity to another transgender person was probably one of the best sexual decisions I've made in my life. Being able to be entirely authentic while in the bedroom made my first sexual experiences with another person quite special and fulfilling.

3. **Plan for it in advance—but keep your plans flexible.** Forget the heat of the moment! You're more likely to have a good time and no regrets if you and your partner have talked things over before the day (or night) itself. Planning can also help you pick a location that's going to be comfortable for you (not squeezed into a car, or in an unlocked room where your roommate might walk in on you).

   Avoid the temptation to pretend you've had intercourse before—it'll work far better if your partner knows this is your first time. We've actually done polls of heterosexual guys in our audiences, asking if they wanted to know whether it was first-time intercourse for the person they were about to have sex with. Nearly unanimously they raise their hands to say yes. Then, we ask why. If it's a random hookup and it's not intended to be deeply meaningful, why do you care? Guys always say that whether it's a hookup, a relationship, or something in between, they'd like the chance to make doubly sure they're checking in, being gentle, and doing what they can to make their partner's first time a positive experience.

If you're expecting to have intercourse for the first time on a special date like your wedding night, Valentine's Day, or your birthday, keep in mind that it's okay if things don't come together, so to speak, as you had envisioned. You or your partner may have had too much to drink, you may be exhausted, or something else may have changed your plans. Losing your virginity on the second day of your honeymoon or the day after Valentine's Day is just as sexy.

We were both virgins, and it was about 20 degrees outside, so it wasn't really "optimal." We were just two horny teenagers. He got off, but I was too uncomfortable.

I was told by everyone around me that it would hurt and be uncomfortable. Instead, it felt wonderful! My partner and I were so comfortable with each other, we just did what felt good, making sure to ask each other what we were feeling/thinking and what we enjoyed. Not bad for a first time experience for both of us.

4. **Don't be drunk.** We're not the preachy, finger-wagging types, but on this topic study after study finds the same thing: People who say their first intercourse was pleasurable tend to be ones who didn't drink before the big event. They feel more sensation, communicate better, are more likely to use a condom correctly, and best of all, they remember what happened the next day.

I was drunk and it hurt a lot, even though I was drunk. I did not have an orgasm although my partner wanted me to, so we kept at it. I remember that I wanted to stop but kept going because it was important to him that I had an orgasm. But I didn't.

I was drunk at the time and don't remember too much, other than it was very rushed, and I was very disappointed.

Obviously, it's one thing to have a glass of wine or a beer with a partner you know and trust before you try first-time penetration, especially if you already have your birth control plans worked out and you're all set with safer sex supplies. That's a very different scenario than getting smashed, hooking up with a stranger, and hoping for the best.

5. **Keep your expectations down to earth.** Having intercourse may or may not go smoothly the first time. It may or may not feel good from the start. Expecting first-time sex to be sparkling perfection is a recipe for a serious letdown. It's far better to be realistic—and perhaps pleasantly surprised.

> *It hurt pretty damn bad. And I was slightly disappointed. In my life, sex was something forbidden, something I wasn't supposed to do, so of course in my head I thought, if it's forbidden and worth waiting for, it must feel really good, like the best feeling in the whole world. And the first time, it definitely was not what I thought it was going to be. Although it was rather nice.*

> *From what I read in books and so on, I thought it would either hurt or be the best experience ever. It didn't hurt since I was comfortable with the guy and ready, but it was over really fast and kind of a disappointment.*

6. **Be comfortable with fingers already.** If you find it uncomfortable or painful to have a finger or two (your own or your partner's) inside your vagina in a sexual situation, then that's your first assignment. That can help get you used to the sensation of having something

inside your vagina. Get to a point where having a finger inside is comfortable for you before trying to insert a penis. Wet your finger with saliva, water, or lube before inserting it.

Experiment first with fingering because it loosens the hymen and allows your partner to find places that feel good to you inside. This will also help to take away some of the mystery of sex, making it seem less intimidating. I lost my cherry during fingering over several occasions. Then, having sex for the first time felt wonderful, instead of the painful experience my friends had warned me of.

7. **Use birth control.** If one person's body has eggs and one person's body makes sperm, then yes, you can get pregnant the first time. Unless you're absolutely positive neither of you could have an STI or HIV (for instance, you've both been tested, or neither of you has ever been sexually active with anyone else), you should be using condoms as birth control or in addition to another kind of birth control. Condoms plus a backup method like contraceptive film, foam, or inserts—all sold near the condoms in most pharmacies and supermarkets—are a highly effective combo to prevent pregnancy. Condoms plus a hormonal method of birth control (pill, patch, ring, implant, shot, hormonal IUD) are even more effective, as are condoms plus a nonhormonal IUD.

8. **Get good and turned on first.** Being aroused before you try penetration isn't just a bonus—it's a requirement for making intercourse comfortable. Spend plenty of time kissing, making out, enjoying each other. Oral sex can be good if you like it. Having an orgasm before you try penetration can work well too.

I wish I had known that it's much more enjoyable with more foreplay. I had barely any foreplay the day I lost my virginity, but that really does make a difference.

Being relaxed is the key to enjoying sex. Engage in foreplay and wait until your body signals you to move on.

9. **Use lube.** Even if you're already wet, and even if your partner's wearing a lubricated condom, add more water-based or silicone lube on top of the condom. Slippery is a very good thing when it comes to penetration.

   It started out passionate and slow on the couch with oral sex, then we moved to the bedroom and continued to be very sweet. He was a pretty large fellow in terms of penis size, and I was terrified. But he was really gentle and took things slowly. We used lots of lubricant and good, sturdy condoms. It didn't hurt at all. We even got crazy with it and sort of did it all over the house: in the bathroom, the shower, the sink, the table. It sort of just spread everywhere. It was incredible.

   It was hard because we were worried about getting caught, and I was too dry—I wish I had known about and been comfortable using lube!

10. **Your partner should definitely *not* plan to "deflower" you in one mighty, powerful thrust.** Ouch! It's also okay if you don't "go all the way" in one session. If it's not feeling comfortable, get as far as it feels okay, and try again another time.

    If your partner is on top, ask them to insert their penis just the smallest amount, then stop, make sure that feels okay, then push in just a teeny bit farther and stop again. You'll want to kiss and breathe along the way, and let your bodies relax together. When you say it's okay, your partner can push in a little farther or do an out-in motion of pulling out and then pushing in just a little farther than last time. You should be in charge here: You decide when it's okay to go farther, when to rest, where to stop. You should discuss this approach in advance, using phrases like "really slow and gentle," and "I heard it would be more comfortable for me if we…" It can also work well for you to be on top: in that position, it's even easier for you to control the depth and speed of penetration.

Breathe! Have your partner go in slowwwly, maybe a half inch at a time, and make him wait until you tell him to go again. Basically play red light/green light until he's in, and then wait a few minutes before he moves again, going very slowly the whole time!

For me, it wasn't the romance you see in the movies. It was me and my boyfriend. In a dorm. Having awkward sex. And his penis didn't fit inside me for a long time. It took us a while to figure it all out.

11. **Don't expect an orgasm through first-time intercourse.** Although it certainly isn't impossible, don't be disappointed if there's no O for you the very first time. One study published in the *Journal of Sex Research* found that only 7 percent of cisgender women had an orgasm their first time. Intercourse—like all sexual skills—tends to feel more pleasurable for both partners as you get better at it.

It was completely different than I expected. First of all, it didn't hurt at all. I was always told it would hurt horribly, but it didn't at all, although I was really sore for the next few days. Second, it was a serious disappointment. People don't tell you it takes practice. They make it seem like orgasms happen every time (even when you have no idea what you're doing).

12. **Have a sense of humor.** If you expect your first time to be flawless, you'll probably be disappointed. But if you're ready to enjoy each other, laugh together at unexpected glitches, and work out the fine points, eventually, you'll have a memorable, stress-free experience regardless of exactly what happens.

> *Sex is always full of mistakes even if you've been with the same person for years. Make the best out of those funny bedroom mistakes.*

> *I thought it would be extremely painful, and it was not, but it was not necessarily pleasurable either. I remember laughing a lot.*

6

G Marks the Spot
The G-Spot and Squirting

A flyer in the dorm lobby caught Marshall's eye. He had just returned to his dorm late one night in his first year of college. Printed in a basic Times New Roman font, it read simply, "How to Female Ejaculate," with the next day's date, a time, and a location. There was no other information on the flyer. Marshall stared at the sign to be sure he was reading it correctly. There was no question: The topic was female ejaculation, and there was some kind of event taking place on campus the following night. By the time he came through the lobby on his way to breakfast the next morning, the flyer was gone.

Later that day, Marshall arrived at the lecture hall where the event was scheduled to take place and was surprised to discover it packed with people. The lights dimmed, and a sexily dressed, curly-haired blond woman, Deborah Sundahl, stepped onto the stage. "I'm going to show you something that will *blow your mind*," she announced. Sundahl started the video, and a larger-than-life image of thighs and a vulva appeared on the screen behind her. Suddenly, a clear stream of liquid shot out from between the legs on the screen. The crowd of students gasped and then erupted into amazed murmurs. Sundahl then proceeded to give an educational lecture on the subject. Who knew this would turn out to be one of the more professionally relevant lectures of Marshall's college career!

I ♥ ORGASMS

Nowadays, "squirting" porn is most people's first introduction to the idea that a person with a vagina could ejaculate. This is true even for vagina-owners who have themselves ejaculated. When we asked them whether they experienced it personally or saw it in a video first, the majority had seen it in porn before experiencing it themselves. Porn is certainly great for normalizing that squirting exists; without this knowledge it can be quite surprising if it happens to you! Porn even helped bring squirting into the mainstream. But the squirting in porn can also be misleading as to what typical real-life ejaculation looks like.

Porn is just the tip of the iceberg when it comes to confusion around squirting. The fact that the fluid comes from the urethra leads many a young, accidental squirter to fear that they peed the bed during sex. One woman told us she was so terrified of this sensation of needing to pee that she literally leapt from the bed every time she could feel herself nearing this arousal peak and dashed down the hall to the bathroom. She described it as a highly unsatisfying way to end every sexual encounter!

In fact, there are lots of differences between squirt and urine. Yes, it comes out of the same hole, the urethra, but that's also true for people with a penis, who pee and ejaculate (two different substances) from the same hole (the urethra).

The confusion even reaches into the professional world, where it's debated in medical journals and at sexuality conferences. In this chapter we'll dive into this complex fountain of knowledge and dry off with some Q&A on the other side. Ejaculation for vagina-owners isn't a sign of something going wrong, like wetting the bed, but rather a sign of sexual pleasure and release. Once it's understood, it's an experience that many vagina-owners and their partners celebrate rather than fear.

Ejaculating is probably the best part of sex for me. I wish it happened every time, but then I'd have a lot more laundry to do.

My partner ejaculated while I was performing oral sex on her (along with vibrator penetration), so I was really close to her vagina at the time. It was the most beautiful and sexiest thing I had ever seen.

I did it to myself [made myself ejaculate] a few months ago. It felt great and I was completely amazed that my body could do that! It was like learning I could fly—I felt incredibly alive and powerful, as cheesy as that sounds.

I actually discovered female ejaculation when I was a teenager. I was talking on the phone with this boy that I had been attracted to for years. One thing led to another and we both began talking dirty to each other. I will never forget it. I had my first female ejaculation in a tie-dye beanbag! And I remember freaking out and telling him I had to get off the phone because I had no idea what had just happened! I thought I had peed everywhere! But then it happened after that—a lot. I found out that I'm a regular "squirter" and that I can do it over and over again. While I was really insecure about it at first, I actually came to enjoy it a lot because it really turned my partners on. Now I absolutely love it. It's like I get this really hot sensation all over my body. My legs start to tingle, my toes curl, my back arches, and then it just bursts out and I shake all over. Sounds almost like a seizure, huh? But then afterwards is the best part: I'm so incredibly relaxed and I feel weightless. AMAZING.

What's in a Name?

FOR YEARS, WHEN audience members would ask us about "squirting," we would correct them by saying, "Squirting is the porn name, but the technical term for it is female ejaculation." Well, times have changed. We've come to love the term *squirting* because it's an inclusive, widely understood term that refers to a person with a vagina ejaculating. By comparison, the words *female ejaculation* aren't as good a fit for a trans masculine or nonbinary person who squirts.

However, you'll also read on pages 198–199 that some researchers draw a distinction between what they call squirting and female ejaculation, clouding the waters a bit. In this chapter, we'll sort through all this, and in the end you can decide what you want to call it. Or you can just call it "fun"!

First Things First: The G-Spot

TO UNDERSTAND EJACULATION and squirting, you need a working knowledge of the G-spot because G-spot stimulation is the activity most likely to lead to squirting. Plus, G-spot stroking feels great to some people with a vagina regardless of whether they ejaculate.

Unlike the sensitive parts of the clitoris on the outside of the body, the G-spot is entirely inside the vagina. It's about two to three inches inside, toward the front wall of the vagina.

Are you with us so far? If so, great, because here's where things get a little bumpy. What does the G-spot feel like? Well, it depends on who you ask. Here are a few of the top hits if one were to search online for the answer to that question:

I ♥ ORGASMS

"Raised or bumpy"

"Puffier, harder, bumpier, or ridged"

"Kind of like an orange peel"

"A wrinkly soft peach pit"

"A bean shape"

"Soft or spongy"

"Rather like the roof of the mouth"

Good grief! Does it feel like an orange peel or a bean? Hard or soft? Wait, a *soft* peach pit?

Here's what we've concluded from our research, including the collected hands-on data from folks who have spent a lot of time with fingers inside vaginas: Don't worry about what it feels like to the fingertips, because in a lot of cases it just feels like the rest of the side of the vagina—not particularly distinctive in a way that it can be identified by touch. Instead, focus on the vagina-owner's feelings of pleasure. Most people who enjoy having their G-spot touched say the sensation is quite different from clitoral stimulation.

G-spots usually respond most to firm, massaging pressure, which is why it was long believed that vaginas lacked nerve endings. In the 1950s, when pioneering sex researcher Alfred Kinsey and his colleagues tested the sensitivity of different areas of vulvas and vaginas, they used an instrument like the tip of a cotton swab to touch gently. Not surprisingly, they found vaginas, including their G-spot, generally not responsive to such gentle touch. If they'd tried the deeper pressure of a massaging finger, many of their study subjects likely would have responded quite differently.

Most people with a sensitive G-spot say they enjoy a "come hither" type motion, with fingers curling forward against the front wall of the vagina. If you're looking for the G-spot, let pleasure be your guide. If you're in the vicinity of where you think your G-spot might

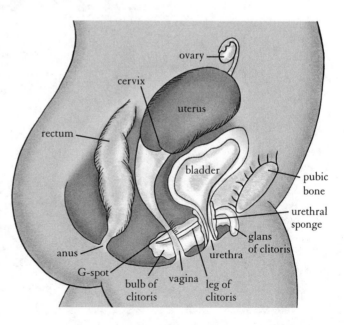

be, and it feels really good to be touched, then congratulations, you've found the G-spot! If you're experimenting with stimulation in that part of your vagina, and you're not finding anything that feels good, that's perfectly normal too. It's normal

What's Your Relationship with Your G-Spot?

MOST RESEARCH STUDIES have found that about two-thirds of people with a vagina find the G-spot area to be sexually sensitive for them. We asked our survey respondents with a vagina how they felt about their G-spot. Here's the breakdown of their answers.

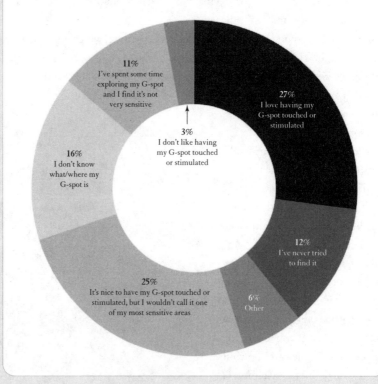

11%
I've spent some time exploring my G-spot and I find it's not very sensitive

3%
I don't like having my G-spot touched or stimulated

27%
I love having my G-spot touched or stimulated

16%
I don't know what/where my G-spot is

12%
I've never tried to find it

25%
It's nice to have my G-spot touched or stimulated, but I wouldn't call it one of my most sensitive areas

6%
Other

I ♥ ORGASMS

to have a G-spot that's really sensitive, equally normal to have one that doesn't really feel like anything, and everywhere in between. Researchers find that the number of nerve endings and amount of arousal tissue in this part of the body vary tremendously from person to person.

Who Put the G in G-Spot?

IN THE LATE 1970s, sex researchers Beverly Whipple and John Perry learned of a sensitive area inside the vagina that could induce ejaculation if stimulated. Researching further, Whipple and Perry discovered that gynecologist Ernst Gräfenberg, a refugee from Nazi Germany living in New York City, had written about this area in a journal article in 1950, but that this anatomical fact had mostly been forgotten during the intervening years. Although the area had also been written about centuries earlier, Whipple and Perry decided to name what they were studying the "Gräfenberg spot," or the G-spot, in honor of the first modern doctor to describe it. The 1982 book *The G Spot* by Perry, Whipple, and their colleague Alice Kahn Ladas sold over a million copies, turning "G-spot" into a household word.

Gräfenberg, who died in 1957, would probably be shocked to realize this one journal article would be the source of considerable posthumous fame. In his own time, he was the chief gynecologist at a hospital in Berlin and best known for designing and creating his own type of intrauterine device (IUD), a form of birth control, in the 1920s. He was the first inventor of an IUD who actually tracked how effective his device was at preventing pregnancy in his patients, and the results were impressive. Unfortunately, the Gräfenberg ring, a relatively primitive device by today's medical standards, was also associated with pelvic inflammatory disease in his patients. Then, the Nazis banned all birth control, which ended all further research.

Nonetheless, when it came to finding the G-spot, Gräfenberg knew he was onto something: "An erotic zone always could be demonstrated on the anterior wall of the vagina," he wrote. "Even when there was a good response in the entire vagina, this particular area was more easily stimulated by the finger than the other areas of the vagina."

Nowadays, we have a much deeper understanding of what's going on in that part of the body, thanks to the research of Whipple and others. The erectile tissue that makes up the G-spot is actually an internal part of the clitoris, part of the same network of interconnected tissue and nerve endings (see the diagram on page 191). The tissue wrapped around the urethra is called the urethral sponge, and as arousal builds, this spongy tissue becomes engorged with blood. Within the urethral sponge are thirty to forty tiny paraurethral glands, the equivalent of the prostate in people with a penis. These produce the fluid of ejaculation, especially when they're stroked and stimulated. During ejaculation, this fluid flows from the glands through ducts into the urethra, and then out of the body.

Meeting Big G

AS WITH ANY sexual exploration, you'll have a better time finding your G-spot if you approach it as an enjoyable, relaxing new adventure rather than a frantic search for a lost item, as though you misplaced your phone or your keys. (Come to think of it, the people who designed the Find My app should consider adding G-spot to the list of devices people could locate using the app. SO USEFUL!) This exploration works best if you're already somewhat sexually aroused. Once you're settled into a comfortable position, gently slide one or two fingers inside your vagina with your palm facing upward, toward your belly button. Push your finger inside your vagina as far as it will comfortably go, and curling it slightly, slowly pull your finger back toward the opening. (If you have long nails or this doesn't feel comfortable, there are also sex toys designed just for this motion. See page 236.) Pay close attention to the sensations as you move your finger along the wall of your vagina that faces your belly button. Experiment with:

○ **The pressure:** Does it feel better if you push really hard against the wall of the vagina or just lightly touch it?
○ **The location:** Does it feel most sensitive when your finger is all the way inside, near the entrance to your vagina, or somewhere in the middle?
○ **The speed:** Is there more sensation when you move firmly and slowly, or do you prefer quick movement?

Also notice the curve of your finger or fingers against your vagina, which for many people is the key ingredient to making this work. You're essentially massaging your vaginal wall, and your goal is to refine your technique to zero in on the movement and touch you find most pleasurable.

Having fun? Good! Wrist getting tired? Say it ain't so! Some find G-spot self-stimulation tiring for the hand or wrist because of the curve involved. If you have a partner, they can be a wonderful assistant to this project. If you recline in bed, your partner can sit or kneel between your legs, giving them comfortable access to your G-spot without tiring either of you out. Have your partner use the same finger techniques described in the previous paragraph. Here's your chance to practice giving your partner really clear, explicit feedback about what feels good and what doesn't. Some couples make it into a game, saying "hot" if the fingers are in the perfect spot, "cold" if they're far from the mark, and "warmer" and "cooler" to provide encouragement and redirection along the way.

In lieu of (or in addition to) a partner, sex toys designed for G-spot stimulation can be another ingredient for a good time, and sometimes easier on the hand and wrist. Read more about these on page 236. Although fingers and toys often provide the most direct G-spot stimulation, there's information about intercourse positions most likely to pleasure the G-spot in Chapter 5. Quick hint: Gräfenberg said doggie style works great; missionary, not so much. (For the record, he described those positions in the parlance of his time: "the lady does lay on her back" and "intercourse from the back of the woman...with the woman in knee-elbow or shoulder position.")

For most people with a vagina, G-spot stimulation is the sexual activity most

The Outer Route to the G-Spot

YOU CAN FEEL the back side of your own G-spot without even putting a finger inside your vagina. Here's how: First, find your pelvic bone, the hard bony area at your lower abdomen, just above the shaft of your clitoris. Inch your fingers up your pelvic bone (toward your belly button) until the bone ends, and you feel the soft flesh of your lower belly. If you push in firmly there—the soft area just above your pubic bone—you may feel a somewhat sensitive area. That's the other side of the erectile tissue that makes up your G-spot. The instructors of a Body Electric sexuality class taught Dorian that they called this spot "the back door to heaven." Pushing in that area is unlikely to be enough to catapult you over the edge to an orgasm. But for some it's an erogenous zone and a bit of added pleasure while masturbating or having partnered sex, and in addition to or instead of internal G-spot stimulation.

likely to lead to ejaculation. Some ejaculate without G-spot stimulation, though, and others find G-spot stimulation really pleasurable in its own right, but haven't found that it leads to ejaculation for them. There are plenty of people with a vagina who just don't find their G-spot particularly pleasurable to massage at all, and that's perfectly fine too.

Sex Tip for Partners: Some Pointers on "Fingering"

BASED ON SNIPPETS of conversation they overheard in the schoolyard and on the backs of school buses, many young people have heard that when a girl invites you to touch her below the waist, what you're supposed to do is "finger her." This unfortunate term has led generations of youth astray, revealing them to be inexperienced lovers and disappointing their partners. Good fingering technique does *not* involve inserting one, two, or as-many-as-you-can-fit fingers into a vagina and quickly thrusting them all the way in and out. Although some people with a vagina might enjoy this practice, most will scrunch their face in displeasure. Likewise, the "fingering" featured in porn is often much rougher and more aggressive than most vagina-owners would like it.

Should your fingers be so lucky as to have direct access to a vagina-owner's privates, first, consent is key (as it is with any partnered sexual activity). With your finger nearby or gesturing in the vicinity of where you're interested in heading, you can ask quietly, "Is this okay?" Suspend operation if you get any response other than a positive one!

Once you confirm you're on the same page, locate the clitoris and spend lots of quality time there, teasing and caressing it and all around the vulva, as described on pages 64–65. After plenty of time there, check in again to be sure your partner wants your finger inside. If you get the green light, note whether you feel any dryness or friction at the opening, and if so, wet your finger first with saliva or lube.

Once inside, casually commence G-spot stimulation, using the techniques described earlier in this chapter. Note that some vagina-owners may prefer your finger to do something else—or not move at all—rather than stimulate the G-spot.

Try a few different things, and ask your partner what feels good. And don't forget to trim your nails before you start! (Or if you love your acrylics, see our advice about gloves and cotton on page 287.)

Start at the clitoris and then work with both the clitoris and G-spot. A lot of the guys I've been with have just started right away fingering me and not even paying attention to the clitoris, which is a major letdown for me.

Unless your partner explicitly encourages or invites these digital behaviors, the three things to avoid are thrusting in and out with speed and force; pulling your finger all the way outside the vagina and then jamming it back in again; and trying to push in as many fingers as you can at once, as though you were trying on a glove.

Despite the confusion about the best fingering technique, don't overlook fingers' massive potential for pleasure.

I love hands! They're so versatile and sensitive. My advice would be, don't be too rough, find out whether I just want to be filled with fingers or whether I want you to move them around, touch me the way you see me touch myself, and use lube!

Gentle is key. Clean hands are a must. But mostly go really slow at first and make sure you are reading your partner like she was the instruction manual to some really cool, really expensive, really fragile gizmo. Basically, pay attention.

Squirt First, Ask Questions Later

FOR MOST VAGINA-OWNERS who have the ability to squirt, lots of G-spot stimulation is what they need to get there. (Some can ejaculate simply from clitoral stimulation, too, though this is less common.) Because squirting isn't a topic in the typical high school sex ed curriculum, it's left a lot of vagina-owners confused when they either accidently discover their own ability or see it in porn.

Porn can be particularly misleading as to what real-life squirting looks like because, like everything in porn, its goal is to be as dramatic as possible for the camera. Porn squirting scenes often involve vigorous G-spot or clitoral stimulation with copious amounts of fluid shooting from the urethra, often traveling considerable distance toward the camera, sometimes in multiple directions at once.

We asked our survey respondents who had ejaculated themselves and also seen squirting porn what they thought the differences were. It was an open-ended question, so they could write whatever they wanted. A full 53 percent of them commented about how the amount of liquid, the intensity, or the degree to which it dramatically shoots out was quite different.

In porn, it's like a waterfall. In real life, it's more like a babbling brook.

Mine wasn't as dramatic, not as forceful. I wasn't even aware I had done it until my partner told me.

For me it kind of gushes out. Sometimes a little, sometimes a lot. It never sprays out in a rainbow-like arch like they show in porn.

So, what *are* they doing in porn? The short answer is, it probably depends on the video. Some porn stars openly admit to peeing when they're being filmed for a "squirting video." Some videos use douches to fill the star's vagina with water just before filming. Some may really be squirting. We've heard other theories, unsubstantiated, about possible special effects. In the end, it doesn't really matter. Porn isn't real life. If you or your partner squirt, chances are good that it won't look like porn's gushing waterfalls and rainbow arches. And if it does, that's normal too:

My experience is porn-like. When it happens, I squirt cups of ejaculate at a time—it goes everywhere, we're all drenched, it's rather climactic for everyone, and others seem to really enjoy it.

What the Research Says

SCIENTIFIC UNDERSTANDING ABOUT squirting has advanced considerably since the first edition of this book—yet still has a long way to go. Meta-analyses have

I ♥ ORGASMS

been published in medical journals in recent years, one analyzing sixty-three studies published between 1950 and 2017, the other analyzing forty-four studies published between 1889 and 2019. By identifying similar conclusions established by multiple different research teams in different ways, these summaries of the research provide a much clearer understanding of the current state of scientific understanding about squirting. Here are the major conclusions:

There are likely two distinct fluids. Apparently squirting isn't just one thing—it's two different things! Although this makes it more confusing to wrap one's mind around this subject, it also explains why different people who squirt sometimes seem to be having such vastly different experiences. ("There's so much liquid that it soaks through several folded towels!" vs "It seems like maybe a tablespoon or two." "It's clear" vs "It's milky.")

In this chapter, we've been using *squirting* and *female ejaculation* to mean the same thing. We mostly choose *squirting* as the more inclusive word. However, the scientific literature increasingly uses those two terms to describe two different fluids. Most people have one or the other, or both combined. To help you sort out the differences, we made you a handy chart!

Based on responses to our survey, "ejaculation" is the more common experience. This thicker, milkier fluid has a lot in common with the semen produced by people with a penis, and like that semen, it contains a lot of PSA (a biomarker often used to test for prostate cancer). It's one of the ways in which the body of people assigned male at birth and those assigned female at birth are more similar than they are different, just as people of all genders have nipples.

I didn't realize I was ejaculating at first, because it was always a small amount of liquid, and not as forceful as some of the female ejaculation I'd heard of before. But after learning more, I realized that I was ejaculating! For me, it's a small amount of liquid and comes only after a large amount of sensation.

Because of its quantity and watery nature, "squirting" seems more similar to what's in porn. Ultrasounds reveal that, unlike ejaculate, squirting fluid is stored in the bladder before it gushes out. Testing finds that it does have some similarities to urine. But people who have experienced it consistently say it doesn't seem to be pee—it doesn't smell like pee and it's not yellow. (We all know that when someone

Squirting, Gushing, Ejaculating: What's What?

	FEMALE* EJACULATION	SQUIRTING (A.K.A. "GUSHING")
What does it look like?	Thicker, milky, more similar to semen from a penis	Thin, watery, clear
How much?	A small amount (less than a teaspoon to a few tablespoons)	A tablespoon to ½ cup or more (looks and feels like a large amount of liquid)
What hole does it come out of?	The urethra	The urethra
Where does it come from inside the body?	Skene's glands inside the urethral sponge	In most cases, the bladder—but characteristics like color and smell make it quite different than urine
How well do scientists understand it?	Fairly well. Many research studies now provide quite detailed information about this.	Not that well. Lots of questions remain and research continues.

* Although the scientific literature uses the word *female*, a person of any gender identity who has a vagina could have this experience.

wets the bed, you can smell it!) One other mystery about this fluid is that vagina-owners in research studies can pee in the lab and have an ultrasound confirm that their bladder is empty. Then, although they were not drinking unusual quantities of liquid, when they masturbate, the bladder rapidly fills with a large quantity of fluid, which they can "squirt" (some studies used the word *gushing*) not long after they had emptied their bladder of urine. What is this mystery fluid? For the time being, no one knows for sure.

If Squirt Smells Like Pee

IT IS POSSIBLE to have "urinary incontinence" during sex. Urinary incontinence, peeing when you don't want or intend to, is a pretty common experience affecting 20 to 40 percent of all adults with a vagina. If a fluid comes out of you and it looks and smells like pee, then it may very well be pee. Most of the time people who experience this also have urinary incontinence at other times during the day, not just during sex, so it doesn't come as a huge surprise to see it happening.

If you find your squirt seems a lot like pee, it's up to you to decide how to think about it. Sadly, some people unnecessarily avoid partnered sex out of shame and embarrassment, but lots of partners don't care. A bit of pee doesn't need to be a big deal, much in the same way sex doesn't need to stop just because you happened to queef. Urine is mostly sterile.

And, of course, there's a sizeable number of people who enjoy "watersports," meaning sex play that involves pee. When it comes to peeing during sex, those partners say, "Bring it on!" But even if seeing pee isn't your partner's idea of a sexy time, given the choice of no sex versus dealing with a little pee in the mix, most would happily accept the trade-off. If it's an ongoing issue, you can decide to have sex in the shower. Or just put down towels and wash them after sex!

There are also medical treatments available. Working with a pelvic floor physical therapist can be quite effective.

Squirting Q & A

Do squirting and orgasm happen at the same time?

For most people with a vulva who ejaculate/squirt, yes, orgasm and ejaculation happen at the same time. This isn't the case for everyone, though—some vulva-owners ejaculate/squirt some time before their orgasm, or shortly after, or they ejaculate/squirt without having an orgasm at all. And, of course, lots of people with a vulva have orgasms without ever ejaculating/squirting in their lives. As always, sexual diversity rules!

It usually happens when I have an orgasm. The stronger the orgasm, the more likely ejaculation is to happen. It is sometimes a strong quick spurt, and sometimes it's a slower trickle, depending on the level of exertion I've used to get to the orgasm.

For me when I ejaculate it's a different feeling than an orgasm. It's hard to explain. My body feels great all over, intense and kind of gushy, for lack of a better word. It's not the same shuddering, vibrating feeling I feel when I have an orgasm. Ejaculating is different every time. It's sometimes well before I have an orgasm, while I'm having one, or just before.

What's the difference between "getting wet" (lubricating) and ejaculating/squirting?

When a person with a vagina becomes aroused, the vaginal walls sweat, so to speak, much in the same way that your skin sweats in hot weather. The liquid, or transudate, is a colorless component of blood that's secreted through the walls of the vagina. That's different from these fluids that come out the urethra.

Given that some people's vagina gets very wet when aroused, and some ejaculations are quite small, in some cases it can be tough to tell the difference. It can be tricky to hold your phone in selfie mode, attempting to see exactly which hole the liquid is coming from. It's also common for small quantities of ejaculate to go unnoticed. If you find yourself puzzling over whether you ejaculated or just got really wet, a few key differences are that lubrication often happens gradually, is produced inside the vagina, and can start quite early in the arousal process. Ejaculation, on the other hand, happens all at once, comes from the urethra, and usually (though not always) takes place around the time of an orgasm.

Do people with a vulva like ejaculating? Is it better than just having an orgasm?

Some love the feeling of release with ejaculation and say it's fun to be able to see physical evidence of their orgasm coming out of their body (similar to the way many penis-owners seem to think ejaculating is pretty cool to do). Others say the experience is just different, neither better nor worse, than having a nonejaculatory orgasm. There's no research evidence to suggest that people with a vulva who ejaculate have better orgasms, or are more sexually satisfied, than those who don't.

Having an orgasm without ejaculating is less pleasurable for me than having one while ejaculating. It also makes for a more intense orgasm.

The feeling of ejaculating is good but not as good as a clitoral orgasm.

I like having an orgasm without ejaculating. I can concentrate on how it feels and not the mess I'm making or that I'm lying in a puddle.

Sometimes I have stronger orgasms when I'm not ejaculating and sometimes it's the opposite. I don't see a huge difference, but usually an orgasm that makes me ejaculate feels better than when I'm not ejaculating.

Some trans masculine folks who are able to squirt find the experience thrilling, and reminiscent of cis men's ejaculation:

Ejaculating orgasms are always really great if I'm feeling dysphoric about my genitals.

Experiencing a partner squirting while you're pleasing them and squirting for a partner have both become delightful surprises and intense pleasures for me.

If you don't already ejaculate, you should feel zero pressure to learn how. If you're curious, sure, give it a try and see whether you can learn. But this does not need to be one more thing on your already overwhelming to-do list ("Get car inspected, do the laundry, call Grandma, learn to squirt"). You can have a fabulous, fulfilling sex life without ever ejaculating.

Can all people with a vulva ejaculate?

Sex experts disagree on this question. Some say that yes, all are capable of learning to ejaculate if they don't do it already. Others say it might be more like rolling your tongue: Some bodies can do it; others can't. Research findings range widely, reporting anywhere from 10 to 68 percent of vagina-owners saying they've ejaculated. (In our survey, 38 percent said they've ejaculated, 44 percent said they haven't, and 19 percent weren't sure.)

Are you sure it's not pee?

The most compelling proof we've read that ejaculate is not pee was an experiment done by a woman curious to figure out the source of her orgasmic expulsions. She was on a medication that turns urine blue, and then proceeded to masturbate, repeating the experiment several times. She would ejaculate on her sheet, and then pee on the same sheet. The pee spots were always deep blue, as expected from the medication. The ejaculation spots either had no color or a faint bluish tinge. A human sexuality professor wrote up the woman's experiments in the *Journal of Sex Research*. Who knew that masturbation could play an important role in advancing science?

If ejaculation is something you'd like to experience, but you're finding yourself fighting the urge to pee, first, be reminded that most people (both vagina- and penis-owners) find it impossible to urinate when they're highly aroused. That's thanks to the Skene's glands for people with a vagina, and the prostate for people with a penis, both of which swell around the urethra when you're aroused. Once you've emptied your bladder (either before sex or by taking a quick bathroom break in the middle of it), decide not to worry about peeing. Give yourself permission to let whatever comes out of your body come out. Put a towel or two on the bed for your own peace of mind. That way, in the highly unlikely event that it's urine and not ejaculate, you can do the same thing you'd do if you had just ejaculated: Put the towels in the washing machine and call it a night!

The first time I did it, I was with my boyfriend. I was terrified, I thought I peed the bed, but he laughed at me and explained what it was. Now it happens all the time when he fingers me, and we just put a towel down ahead of time for me to lie on.

It's very clear, pretty much odorless, sometimes just a little and sometimes a substantial amount, like maybe half a cup of liquid. And after squirting, and possibly a separate orgasm, I'll often get up and still have a full enough bladder to pee, which looks and smells different. My girlfriend and I feel like we've answered the question.

But it feels like I need to pee!

That's very common—as people with a vulva get sexually excited, the spongy tissue surrounding the urethra swells up with blood. This tissue squeezes the urethra and can press against the bladder, too, creating a sensation very similar to the urge to pee. These sensations are totally normal with arousal and can be a sign that you're about to ejaculate.

If you're still feeling nervous about it, you can always be sure you pee before sex, or if the feeling arises, stop what you're doing sexually, go pee, and then return to your sexual activities. If, a short time afterward, you feel a strong urge to urinate, you know you just went, so this time you can be reassured that the fullness you're feeling is ejaculate, not urine. After experiencing this once or twice, you can gain confidence in the source of the sensation so you no longer need to interrupt yourself to visit the loo.

Does taking hormones affect squirting for trans folks?

Taking hormones can affect your experience of squirting, making it easier for some and harder for others. It seems that with most things about the ways bodies work, there's not one set of ways a body will change and respond to hormones shifting.

Testosterone made me drastically more sensitive, and more prone to multiple orgasms and squirting.

I come differently now since I started HRT. I used to squirt all the time, and now I don't.

I want to squirt! How can I make it happen?

The most likely route to that goal (though not the only one) is lots of G-spot stimulation. For most people interested in squirting, the most effective kind of stimulation is with fingers making a "come hither" finger motion, as discussed earlier. A partner or a G-spot-stimulating sex toy can help too. When you feel the urge to pee, and/or while you're having an orgasm, you may want to take the fingers, sex toy, or penis out of your vagina to allow space for the ejaculate to come out, and practice letting go or pushing out the same way you do when you pee. As with so many other aspects of orgasms, having strong PC muscles can make a big difference. Be sure to do your Kegels, as described on pages 34–36, 38.

Penises don't tend to work as well for leading to squirting, perhaps because the stimulation isn't as direct, and perhaps because they tend to block the fluid's ability to come out.

Recently I got divorced, went back to college, and got a new boyfriend. In college I was taking this human sexuality class, and the textbook included some information about female ejaculation. One night during the semester I was taking the class, my boyfriend and I were trying some new things, and I had an orgasm, and I squirted! I'd never done this before, but I was so excited! I was jumping up and down naked in the bedroom, telling him, "It's just like in the textbook! It's just like in the textbook!"

In my early 40s, my girlfriend was putting pressure with her fingers next to my clit, and clear liquid started coming out. I realized I was squirting and relaxed into this possibility more and more over the next few years. I started to get a sense of how to let the squirting happen or even let it build and release sometimes. Now, it might be prompted by playing with my tits, a look, being licked, or penetration, with my girlfriend or solo.

Squirting: Something Old or Something New?

ALTHOUGH EJACULATION FOR vagina-owners is a new concept to many people alive today, it's long been known that people with a vulva had the potential to ejaculate—some cultures even saw ejaculation as healing, sacred, or essential for conception. Ancient Chinese and Indian sexuality texts wrote about it over two thousand years ago. Aristotle, Galen, and other ancient Greek philosophers and scientists examined the subject in detail. Renaissance anatomists documented the existence of glands that produced ejaculate. In sixteenth-century Japan, women used special bowls to catch their own ejaculate, which was believed to have healthy, aphrodisiacal properties. Batoro women in Uganda reportedly teach their young women how to ejaculate before they're considered eligible for marriage—their word for the custom is *kachapati*, which translates to "spray the wall."

Despite all this, the very concept that people with a vulva are able to ejaculate managed to be forgotten for most of the eighteenth and nineteenth centuries, only to be "discovered" all over again in recent decades.

What about the C-spot, the P-spot, and the A-spot?

Are you seeing spots? Sometimes it seems like there's a new one "invented" every month. Here's a quick primer:

○ **C-spot:** Another word for clitoris. Don't let anyone fool you into thinking you're not in the know when they call it the C-spot.
○ **P-spot:** The P stands for prostate, stimulated from inside the anus of people assigned male at birth. See Chapter 11 for more details.
○ **A-spot:** Anterior fornix spot, also known as the AFE-zone (anterior fornix erogenous zone). It's a smooth area just below the cervix, on the front

of a vagina (the same side as the G-spot) but farther up, deeper inside the vagina. Some people find the area quite erotically sensitive; others don't.

Personally, when we follow the directions about where to find the A-spot (did you think we could write a book about orgasm without doing any—*ahem*—hands-on research?), we think it's just another location for the G-spot. Some G-spots are closer to the cervix; others, closer to the entrance to the vagina. But one thing is certain: the discovery of new spots and sex positions grabs attention, scoring clicks.

The reality is, bodies are covered in erogenous zones; it's only a matter of figuring out which places are most sensitive for any particular person. We say, if you discover a new area that feels good to touch, great, enjoy! If your friend has a sensitive spot and you don't have one in that exact same area, there's no need to lose sleep over it—you can likely find plenty of others. Gräfenberg himself couldn't agree more, writing in his original 1950 paper that started all this fuss: "Innumerable erotogenic spots are distributed all over the body, from where sexual satisfaction can be elicited; these are so many that we can almost say that there is no part of the female body which does not give sexual response, the partner has only to find the erotogenic zones." Happy searching!

7

A Golden Era of Sex Toys

From the invention of the wheel to the app that lets you play your phone like a harmonica, humans take pride in our ability to invent and use tools. Never before in human history, though, have there been so many choices of tools whose sole purpose is getting people off. We're living in a golden era of sex toys. It's a great time to be alive!

Like other types of technology, sex toys have been rapidly evolving to meet a greater range of desires for sensation, aesthetics, and sex play. As taboos have faded, toys began appearing on the shelves of mainstream retailers like Walmart and Amazon, as well as at your local drugstore, an aisle or two over from the cough medicine. Growing numbers of independently owned sex toy shops continue to pop up, with gorgeous websites and the kind of stylish interiors that invite you to spend a Friday evening browsing with friends. As a result of all this availability, sex toys have landed in hundreds of millions of bedside drawers worldwide.

Vibrators

VIBRATORS ARE THE monarch of sex toys, essentially vibrating toys for grownups. They come in every shape, size, and style you can imagine, ranging from a little vibrating "bullet" designed to be slipped inside your underwear, to a device the size of a rolling pin. Some vibrators are cleverly disguised as a tube of lipstick, easily kept in a purse in case of an afternoon emergency. Others look like a sleek pendant necklace, unrecognizable for what they are except to those in the know. Some look like bunny rabbits, rubber duckies suited for the tub, tongues, or undulating abstract sculptures. Some are breathtakingly Instagram-worthy art pieces, and others look about as utilitarian as the flashlight you keep around in case the power goes out.

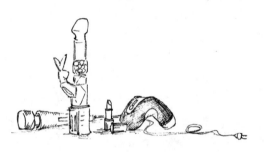

Why do vibrators lead to so many orgasms? It so happens that many clitorises *love* the sensation of vibration. No hand or tongue can maintain the fast, intense, consistent stimulation that a vibe provides—and a vibrator never gets a cramped neck or an aching wrist. For many people, a vibrator is the fastest route to orgasm; for others, it's the only way they can get there. Since it's common for people with a vulva to take longer to come than they'd like, anything that speeds the process is often a welcome enhancement. There's no stereotypical vibrator user either. Some enjoy vibrators to make a great partnered sex life even better; others, to keep them whistling when they're single. Vibrators can be especially welcome after menopause, when orgasms can take longer, since they can take the pressure off partners (and tired hands and fingers).

And science suggests there are health benefits too. Researchers at Indiana University report, "The data indicate that the women who have used vibrators—and particularly those who have done so most recently—experience more positive sexual function in terms of desire, arousal, lubrication, orgasm, and pain." The researchers make clear that the study doesn't address causation: do vibrators actually improve sexual function, or are people who are already doing well more likely to use vibrators? Either way, things are looking good for those who have a collection of vibes!

I had my vibrator for almost a month before I finally had the time to experiment with it. The first time, I stopped before I orgasmed; I think the pleasure kind of shocked me into stillness. It took me a few nights to figure out what I liked and what just didn't work for me. When I finally did orgasm, it was just, like, whoa. My entire body was shaking and I continued to tremble for a few minutes after. This discovery was quite possibly the best thing to happen to me that year. All I could think was, Why haven't I done this before?

The modern vibrator, like so many appliances, followed electricity into the home in the late 1800s. Vibrators were among the first few electrical appliances available to the general public, appearing soon after toasters and nearly a decade before vacuum cleaners and electric irons. By 1900, they were marketed in catalogs for home use—but with no indication of their tremendous benefit to one part of the body in particular. Newspaper advertisements and mail-order catalogs promised women the devices would offer "thrilling, refreshing vibration" and help buyers "realize thoroughly the joy of living." That type of advertising continued for many decades.

The sexual revolution of the 1960s and '70s set in motion today's increasing acceptance of vibrators. Pioneering sex educator and masturbation advocate Betty Dodson started offering workshops on masturbation and recommending the Hitachi Magic Wand, and soon many happy customers, sex therapists, and popular magazines were doing the same. In the ensuing years, it gained an iconic status, hailed as the "mother of all vibrators" and "the most recognizable sex toy on Earth."

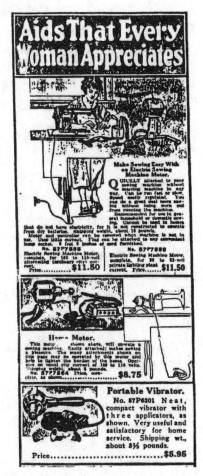

This listing from a 1918 Sears, Roebuck and Company catalog advertises vibrators right underneath the sewing machines.

A Vibrating Tall Tale

IN THE FIRST edition of this book, we reported on the fascinating conclusions of scholar Rachel Maines's book *The Technology of Orgasm*. Maines claimed that from 300 BCE to the 1920s, doctors massaged women's genitals to orgasm as an accepted medical treatment for "hysteria." When the vibrator was invented, Maines said, doctors turned to machines to do the work they used to do by hand, saving them time and effort. It was a major moneymaker since, she wrote, "These patients neither recovered nor died of their condition but continued to require regular treatment." Everyone was so clueless about the clitoris that no one thought of this act as sexual, or so Maines would have had us believe.

Maines's sensational story—women going to doctors week after week for clitoral stimulation sessions—went viral over the course of a decade. The book was widely cited in scholarly literature, has been made into films and a Tony-nominated play, was translated into multiple languages, and has even been cited in court cases. Like many sex educators, we'd been reporting the book's conclusions as fact.

Unfortunately, the tale was too good to be true. It turns out there's no evidence supporting any of it, as professors Hallie Lieberman and Eric Schatzberg painstakingly detail in their journal article, "A Failure of Academic Quality Control: The Technology of Orgasm." Alas, doctors may have invented vibrators, but they weren't running a lucrative side business providing electromechanical hand jobs with them. Lieberman put it best when she wrote in the *New York Times*, "It's time to be honest about our past: doctors didn't invent vibrators because their wrists hurt from rubbing hysterical women's clitorises. They invented vibrators as cure-all devices; those devices ended up curing very little, until our great-great-grandmothers put them toward their highest purpose. The real story isn't as salacious as the myth, but it does have one important thing going for it: it happens to be true."

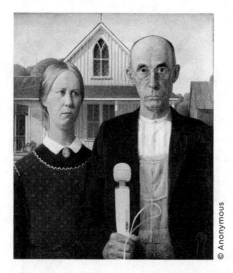

The Magic Wand vibrator has become so iconic that one artist started inserting it into classic works of art like American Gothic. This couple just might start smiling soon.

A standard vibrator like the Magic Wand uses a concept called "rotating unbalance" to do its work. Imagine a motor spinning a small wheel very fast: in the case of the Magic Wand, six thousand revolutions per minute. The wheel is also designed to be slightly off balance and shakes as a result, much like the way a top-loading washing machine vibrates if the clothes inside aren't evenly distributed. That vibration can feel great on a body part like the clitoris that's sensitive to that type of stimulation.

I have a round vibrator that is gentle but has many rhythm settings that are less robotic. I'm demisexual and not having another person to interact with makes masturbation more difficult, so this toy with its asymmetrical rhythms feels more reminiscent of a human's motion.

I find most vibrators too powerful, so I prefer a simple bullet vibe if I'm going to use one at all.

I love a good old wand. I like the dispersed vibration. It vibrates a little slower but with more intensity than a regular vibrator.

But "rotating unbalance" isn't the only way to polish the pearl. The new tech on the block uses air suction designed to mimic the sensation of cunnilingus. A number of companies now sell air-suction "vibrators."

I like using my clitoral suction vibrator. It's quiet and it provides direct stimulation without the buzzy-ness of a vibrator.

How do these kinds of toys work? They're typically a handheld device with a hollow, thimble-size head that fits over the head of the clitoris. The toy then gently blows and sucks air in and out, creating a feeling that's, well, pretty sensational for most clit-owners. They're usually packaged with different size heads and can be adjusted for different levels of intensity.

Where to Get Your Hands on a Vibe

Could a Vibrator Be the Ticket to a First Orgasm?

A FULL 16 percent of the people with a vulva who answered our survey said their first orgasm was from a vibrator. And vibrators were frequently mentioned when we asked our survey respondents what advice they would give to others trying to have their first. Typical suggestions were perhaps best summed up by the person who submitted simply this all-caps advice: "VIBRATORS ARE YOUR FRIEND."

CURIOUS? READY TO give it a whirl—or should we say, a buzz? Sure, you could pick up a vibe at the nearest pharmacy, but there are way more fun—and informative—ways to go about this.

You're particularly in luck if you live in or near a city with a gender-inclusive LGBTQ-friendly sex toy boutique. These stores pride themselves on being warm, inviting spaces that are welcoming to women and LGBTQ people, as well as to cisgender straight men. They aim to stock high-quality, body-safe merchandise—we say, "no, thanks!" to toxins in our nether regions! But their biggest selling point is their staff: knowledgeable people who are comfortable answering questions and offer candid advice without embarrassment to people of all sexual histories, experiences, and backgrounds.

Most of the ones on the list are owned by women, queer-identified folks, and/or people of color, and many offer fun educational workshops on a variety of sexuality topics. It's worth following them on social media or getting on their email list.

Around the United States and the World:

Albuquerque, NM	Self Serve
Atlanta, GA	Liberator Shop
Austin, TX	Q Toys
Baltimore, MD	Sugar
Berkeley, CA	Good Vibrations, Feelmore510
Boston, MA	Good Vibrations
Chicago, IL	Early to Bed
Denver, CO	Awakening Boutique
Edmonton, CA	Traveling Tickle Trunk
Los Angeles, CA	The Pleasure Chest, Cupid's Closet
Madison, WI	A Woman's Touch
Milwaukee, WI	The Tool Shed
Minneapolis, MN	The Smitten Kitten
New Orleans, LA	Dynamo
New York, NY	Babeland, Eve's Garden, Please, Pleasure Chest, Shag
Northampton, MA	Oh My!
Oakland, CA	Feelmore510
Philadelphia, PA	Sexploratorium, Indulgence Boutique
Portland, ME	Nomia Boutique
Portland, OR	She Bop
Provincetown, MA	Toys of Eros
San Francisco, CA	Good Vibrations
Seattle, WA	Babeland
Ventura, CA	Trystology

Berlin, Germany	Other Nature
Cape Town, South Africa	Allure Sensuality Emporium
Halifax, Canada	Venus Envy
Hong Kong	Sally's Toy
London, UK	Sh!
Madrid, Spain	Los Placeres de Lola
Moscow, Russia	G-spot
Ottawa, Canada	Venus Envy
Santiago, Chile	Japi Jane
Sydney, Australia	Max Black
Tokyo, Japan	M's
Toronto, Canada	Come as You Are, Good for Her
Vancouver, Canada	Womyns' Ware, Art of Loving

This list is definitely *not* all-inclusive. New stores pop up every year, and there are now so many great ones out there that it's hard to keep track of them all.

Clearly, we're big fans of the world of sex toy boutiques and always make a point to check out the local one if we're in a new city that has one. We've also enjoyed our time immersed in an entirely different world of toy sales: home sex toy parties. The one we've gotten to know best—though by no means the only player in this field—is Pure Romance. Companies like these have legions of representatives (Pure Romance has 40,000), nearly all women, who sell toys, lingerie, and sensual body products at social gatherings, usually in other women's living rooms. We first found ourselves plunged into this realm when we were hired for several consecutive years to train the representatives of a similar company that was later acquired by Pure Romance. We spoke to a sea of sex-positive, enthusiastic salespeople in a giant convention center ballroom, teaching about sexual pleasure to help them be more effective and better prepared to field their customers' questions. Afterward, the line of consultants eager to stock up on our orgasm book, T-shirts, socks, and buttons always wound farther than we could see.

Since then, we've been impressed by the small groups of consultants we've gotten to know better as we've led workshops at small team retreats. Often, they're educating an entirely different clientele than the ones seeking out sex toys: women who might not have ever imagined adding a toy to their lives until a friend invited them to a home party. Many of the representatives are at-home moms outside urban centers, running part-time businesses while their kids are in school and after they put them to bed at night, selling to others in their towns and social networks. While opening a store takes one kind of bold entrepreneur, discussing orgasms in communities with a rigid no-sex-talk taboo can require its own kind of courageous, business-minded spirit. The parties they lead are unquestionably expanding access to sex toys—and orgasms!

What Kind of Vibrator?

WHETHER YOU'RE CHOOSING your first toy or adding to a sizable collection; whether you buy at a home party, a boutique, the corner store, or an online retailer; here are some factors to consider as you make your selection.

Vibrators come in all different shapes and styles but generally fall into four categories: clitoral vibrators, vaginal/G-spot vibrators designed to be used internally, ones that stimulate both the clitoris and internally at the same time, and ones that are designed for some other body part, like the penis or the prostate.

Clitoral Vibrators

Vibes designed solely for clitoral stimulation can range from a toy smaller than your pinkie finger to a large wand style. It's no surprise they're the top-selling type: they're designed to stimulate the most sensitive body part, and they do a darn good job of it. As one Pure Romance consultant told us, "I'll never forget getting a phone call from a sixty- to seventy-year-old woman who bought a clitoral vibrator from me. She called to thank me for helping her have her first orgasm in her life."

Not only are clitoral vibes easy to use, many people find them nonthreatening, since they're often not phallic-shaped and therefore don't look like they might "substitute" for a penis-owning partner. Some types can even work well for stimulation *during* penetration by a partner.

I have a small vibrator and it's nice to place it on my clitoris or between my labia. It's a sensation I can't produce with my bare hands.

I usually use a vibrator that focuses on the clitoris (which I refer to as my dick/penis). The vibrations on all the area around my dick and my "foreskin" are what feel the best, because direct contact on my dick is too sensitive and can be unpleasant.

My "wand" plugs into the wall for maximum strength vibration. I love that the head is broad, I love that when I use pressure in addition to the vibration it doesn't disturb the vibration at all. I can have an orgasm in under 10 seconds using it.

Vaginal/G-Spot Vibrators

Not everyone needs or wants clitoral stimulation, particularly at the same time as G-spot stimulation. For those with sensitive G-spots, a vibe with a curve designed to reach the G-spot can get the job done. Some people prefer to use a G-spot dildo for this job, a nonvibrating toy designed to fit inside the vagina (more on this later in this chapter). Of course, the vibrating kind gives you both options: turn it on if you're in the mood for vibration, or switch it off and use it as a simple dildo.

I have a curved vibe that hits the G-spot beautifully.

The first time a partner used my G-spot vibe on me, I had an out of body experience!!! So much fun. I couldn't believe it could feel that good. It felt very different from using it on myself.

Dual-Action Vibrators

Dual action vibrators are sometimes called "rabbit vibrators" because of the shape that became iconic after its appearance on an episode of *Sex in the City*. This style of vibrator, with infinite variations, is now made by many different companies. Typically they have a phallic-shaped shaft that can be inserted into the vagina, plus a part that branches off the shaft (often shaped like bunny ears) to provide clitoral stimulation. In the words of a Pure Romance consultant:

> *Women love the clitoral stimulation, but at times crave penetration too. Add the two together? FIREWORKS!*

> *I use a tiny black-and-pink lipstick-shaped vibrator. I wanted one because I wasn't ready for intercourse, but I wanted to experiment to see what I would like.*

> *Mine is blue and looks like an average-sized penis. It's tilted a quarter of the way up to enable the G-spot to be stimulated. I bought it when I was out with some*

What to Consider When Choosing a Vibe

Shape and size	When buying a TV, bigger may be better, but not necessarily with a vibrator. Sometimes the discreetness and portability of a smaller vibe hits the spot perfectly. If you're using it for penetration, consider starting small, but there's also no shame in being a size queen if that's what you enjoy.
Type of vibration	If possible, buy in-person so you can turn it on and hold it in your hand. Try closing your eyes and feeling the different ways it vibrates. Although you can't try before you buy, trust your instincts about whether it piques your interest.

Power	Do you want a wireless vibrator that has a charging stand or USB charger? One that uses standard AAA batteries? Or a corded one that you use while it's plugged in so you can be sure the charge will never run out at a key moment? Vibrators that don't need to be plugged in open up a world of possibilities: In the car? (Not while driving, please.) In the shower? (Get a waterproof one.) Camping? (What better way to enjoy nature?) If you choose the rechargeable kind, think through where your charging station will be, particularly if you live with roommates or have nosy kids in the house.
Price	Like any gadget, brand names can feel overpriced, but knockoffs can break, fail to deliver, or be made of toxic materials. Best advice: take the middle route. Don't break the bank on your first purchase, but do select something you genuinely like and think you'll use. You can always expand your inventory down the road and invest in a fancier model once you know you like the vibrations.
Sound	If your housemate sleeps in the room next door or your dorm room has paper-thin walls, you may want to be sure your vibrator is the strong, silent type. If there's no one to hear your vibe's happy hum, then you have nothing to worry about!
Color and style	What looks like fun to you? A sparkling purple cylindrical smoothie? A vibrator shaped like a well-hung penis? A waterproof curved toy perfect for some rub-a-dub-dub G-spot play? One you'd be proud to display on your shelf as an art piece? Choose one that appeals. You can always diversify down the road.

friends who already had one. I wanted to become more confident with sex. I use it before going out to prevent myself from doing something stupid. I also use it before a nap when I'm really stressed out and to get my mind off things that don't allow me to relax and go to sleep.

My favorite vibrator is small and packs a punch! There's multiple vibrating speeds and patterns. Plus the base is decked out in rhinestones, so it's pretty damn cute.

I have a transparent hot pink basic vibrator. It was a gift, so I didn't pick the color, but it amuses me to no end that it is pink. It makes me feel really girly and normally I'm not a super-girly girl. My mom gave it to me when I was home from college over Thanksgiving break my freshman year, along with a book about masturbation. She wanted to make sure that I was having a good time in college, I guess.

Getting Started with a Vibe

OKAY, SO YOU'VE got your vibrator in hand! Ready for a test drive? How you use it is up to you, based on whatever feels good, but here are a few pointers:

1. Go slow. If your vibe has multiple speeds, start out on low, then experiment to figure out what you like.

2. Play with pressure. Experiment with the lightest touch, firm pressure, and in between.

3. Add a buffer. You may want to put a piece of cloth (e.g., a folded washcloth or some clothing) in between your clit and the vibrator, to soften the intensity.

4. Start with the clitoral area. Even if your vibrator is dual action, consider focusing on the clit at first and going from there. Of course, if you've been eagerly awaiting having it inside you, go for it!

I don't like vibration that's too strong because I'm very sensitive and it numbs me, so my favorite toys are softer ones that vibrate gently. I prefer vibration on my clit and not inside me, so my favorite vibrators are ones that are designed specifically for clit stimulation and not for penetration.

"And It Sends Texts Too"

THERE'S AN APP for everything, including orgasms. Enterprising developers have used mobile phones' built-in vibrating ability to do more than just notify you that your BFF is texting. Most include a few choices of vibration patterns, with in-app purchases for dozens more. It's unlikely these vibrator apps are ever going to be significant competition for the real thing. They might boost sales of waterproof phone cases, though.

And phones aren't the only everyday objects whose vibration can be put to use for other means. We've heard plenty of stories of accidental and intentional orgasms caused by:

- back massagers

- washing machines

- subwoofer speakers playing loud, strong bass

- squiggle pens (We've heard quite a few "first orgasm" stories that involved these battery-operated pens designed to make you write wiggly.)

- electric toothbrushes

- riding lawn mowers

- bicycle seats (there's even a vibrating O-seat sold for this purpose)

- motorcycles

- the gentle rumble of riding in a bus, train, car, or airplane

Trans Masculine Toys

THERE ARE A number of sex toys and types of gear designed specifically with trans masculine people who haven't had bottom surgeries in mind. A number of companies manufacture strokers and sleeves, two types that are among the more popular.

Using toys to jerk off my clit and using different language for it during partnered sex radically transformed orgasms from a chore to a joy.

It was very validating to feel the hand motion of using the sleeve because it's similar to the stroking motion on a penis. I cried the first time I used one because it reaffirmed my sense of feeling like I should have a penis, like a moment of satisfaction in finally feeling what I'd thought I always wanted.

Most of the toys that work best for trans women and femmes aren't actually designed specifically for them, but some companies do have an intentionally expansive and inclusive approach. See page 231 for more.

5. Experiment with different parts of the vulva. While many like to use their vibe directly on their clitoris (or its shaft or side), others get enough stimulation by holding it against their outer lips, or resting their fingers over their clit and using the vibrator to make their fingers vibrate. Experiment with using your vibrator to massage your whole body and all around your genitals.

6. Position yourself. In addition to holding the vibrator in your hand, try resting it on some pillows and then lowering yourself down onto it in a "riding" position.

Or, if your toy is big enough, you can lie back and squeeze it between your thighs, which frees up your hands for other pleasures.

7. Build arousal slowly. If you're climbing toward orgasm faster than you'd like, turn the vibrator off for a bit and then back on again. Seduce yourself. Mix up vibrations with touching your body with your hands, deep breathing, and other mental and physical turn-ons.

Can a Vibrator Desensitize You?

THE MOST-ASKED VIBRATOR question we receive is, "Can a vibrator desensitize you?" There's a widely circulated worry that the intense stimulation a vibrator can provide will numb you, eventually reducing your ability to have an orgasm.

When we put that question to survey respondents who felt like they had used a vibrator enough to have an opinion, 73 percent said they did not think using a vibrator desensitized them, and another 21 percent said they had experienced it as a temporary problem they were able to overcome. Five percent said yes, they thought using a vibrator had desensitized them in a way they found challenging.

Using slightly different language, researchers at Indiana University surveyed two thousand women and asked whether those who had used a vibrator had ever experienced numbness as a side effect. Eighty-four percent said they'd never felt numb, 13 percent said they'd experienced numbness once or a few times, and 3 percent felt numb every time they used their vibrator. Of those who had experienced at least occasional numbness, most said it lasted less than five minutes.

Given these findings, we don't think there's much cause for concern. In the unlikely situation you experience some numbness or loss of sensitivity, take a break. Stop using the vibrator for a while (an hour or a few days will probably do it). In almost all cases, spending some time using your hand or your partner's hand instead of a toy will give your body a breather, and then you'll be free to return to toy use if you want to. There's no evidence that vibrators cause permanent damage or do any lasting harm (and a mountain of evidence that they do a lot of good)!

I started using the vibrator as a garnish instead of the main course, and slowly easing off it until I no longer required it. It also helped to give myself occasional breaks from stimulation if I felt I was becoming desensitized, and usually my sensitivity would return to normal within two or three days.

Another concern you can lay to rest is the idea that you'll get addicted to your vibrator and be unable to come other ways. Not to worry! Most people who use vibrators see them as a way to add variety to their sexual menu, like picking up a pack of peanut butter cup brownies from the supermarket, instead of always buying Ben & Jerry's. Studies of vibrator users find the vast majority still come in other ways.

Even if you find vibrating is your favorite (or only) way to come, that's perfectly okay! No vibrator police will arrive at the door to confiscate your vibrator when you reach a certain age or get married. If a vibrator is what gets your Os flowing better than anything else, you can simply include your vibe in your sex life until the day you die.

If you find that a vibrator's extra-strong sensations are making it harder to tune into a hand or tongue's more subtle sensations the way you used to, no problem. Try retiring your vibrator temporarily so you can recalibrate to mellower stimulation. If you were able to come in other ways before, your body will certainly relearn. If it's never worked for you and still doesn't, that's fine too—many people with a clitoris are in your situation. Of course, don't expect every orgasm to feel the same: orgasms from different kinds of stimulation feel different. For more on changing the way you come, including exploring how to come without a vibrator, see page 102.

All I Want for Christmas Is an Electric Toothbrush

ONE WOMAN SHARED that as a teenager, she asked her parents to get her an electric toothbrush for Christmas. She let them believe she wanted to improve her dental hygiene, but her real plans were a *lot* more fun than cavity prevention.

Babe, I'd Like You to Meet My Vibrator

VIBRATORS LOVE COMPANY! Many vibrator aficionados like the idea of using their vibrator while they're with a partner, but worry how the partner might respond to the idea of making love with a battery-operated "friend" in the mix. Luckily, most partners think vibrator play is sexy. In a study published in the *Journal of Sex Research,* only 10 percent of vibrator owners said their partner was negative or unenthusiastic about it. Many get the concept that if sex is about pleasure, and if vibrators provide lots of it, it's likely to be a great time all around!

Vibration Nation?

WHAT DO GOOGLE searches tell us about interest in sex toys? Here are the top ten countries in terms of the frequency of searches for sex toy words like "vibrator" or "dildo" (in their own language). The numbers indicate the number of searches per one thousand Internet users.

1. Denmark: 118
2. Sweden: 115
3. Greenland: 108
4. United States: 104
5. United Kingdom: 96
6. Netherlands: 88
7. Russia: 87
8. Bulgaria: 86
9. Italy: 84
10. Australia: 82

He was a little wary at first, but because I use a small vibrator that doesn't get in the way, he doesn't mind, and he actually likes trying to coordinate our orgasms to happen at the same time. This wouldn't be possible without the extra stimulation from the toy.

My partner feels that a sex toy would not allow him to perform his "manly duty." He feels that he should be the only one giving me orgasms.

Toys that pleasure both parties are a gift from the gods. And for me, seeing my partner in physical pleasure really heightens my own physical pleasure.

Part of the trick, of course, is how the vibrator-inclined partner broaches the subject. Saying something to the effect of, "Honey, you're such a pathetic lover, I got myself a machine to get the job done right," is not likely to go over well. But if you say, "I think it could be really hot to play with a vibrator together sometime—do you want to try it?" or "I always have the most amazing orgasms when I think of you and use my vibe. Imagine I brought it to the bedroom with us next time and you be there in real life?," a partner is likely to be intrigued. Going vibrator shopping together (in person or online) can help make it a joint project—not to mention being an excellent conversation starter about what sorts of bedroom fun appeal to you. Here's what some of our survey respondents said about using a toy with their partner:

> *My boyfriend actually got out my toy and used it on me. I was ecstatic! I thought it was so awesome that my boyfriend approached it before I could ask him. We still use toys, and he even has some.*

> *My girlfriend and I really enjoy using sex toys together. It allows us to be a little kinky. We're not the most kinky, sex-crazed people, so it's sort of an adventure for us.*

> *Using a sex toy was his idea because his hands get tired (even though he plays guitar).*

> *The act of having my partner use my battery-operated dildo on me was exhilarating, but I could've achieved orgasm better without it.*

> *My partner and I both came to our relationship with a stock of sex toys and carnal knowledge, so we never had to introduce each other to the idea of sex toys. It just seemed a natural part of our sex life.*

When using a vibrator with a partner, either of you can hold it, or you can get one that straps on. Two partners who each have a vagina can rub against the same vibrator, take turns, use one designed for two users, or use two at once. Note that anytime two people's bodily fluids get on a sex toy, there's some risk of STI transmission, including HIV, so take this into consideration when you decide whose fluids will go where.

Cock Rings

VIBRATING COCK RINGS, sometimes called c-rings, attempt to further integrate vibrators into partner play. A cock ring is a ring or cuff designed to be worn around the penis or around both the penis and the scrotum, as close to the body as possible. Most are designed to be quite tight, restricting blood flow so that blood stays in the penis and the erection lasts longer or stays harder.

These kinds of toys have a long history, with some suggesting they may have been used in ancient China and Greece. Adding vibrators to them is a newer addition, with the idea that the attached vibrator could stimulate a partner's clitoris during penetration. Some people with a penis like the sensation of having their penis inside their partner's vagina while a vibrator provides clitoral stimulation. Others like the sensation of having the base of their penis stimulated at the same time as their partner's clit.

Using lube can help to slide a cock ring into position. If your goal is to add vibration during penis-in-vagina sex, cowgirl or reverse cowgirl positions may work best. Like every kind of sex toy, they're not for everyone, and even if it appeals to you, it can take a few tries to find one that fits comfortably. Some prefer the kind that don't vibrate.

I like cock rings: they keep my boyfriend harder longer and some of them have little bumps on them that stimulate my clitoris. We got ours from a local sex shop—it glows in the dark. We got it to try to add some variety to the game.

I joke it turns your partner into a human vibrator! It will get you off AND make you breakfast!

Since getting bottom growth I have been very keen on receiving blow jobs, using cock rings and pumps to make my genitals bigger. These methods give me huge gender euphoria!

App-Controlled Vibrators: The Next Frontier

REMOTE- AND APP-CONTROLLED vibrators move the toy's controls for speed, rhythm, and intensity from the vibe itself to your hands or your partner's. Some of these toys rely on a remote control that comes with the toy, but the trend is to sync your toy with an app and control it from a phone. App-linked toys can be controlled with equal ease by the partner in bed next to you, your long-distance beau on the other side of the world, or some stranger you just met on the Internet. The choice is yours! Often, couples trade off whose hands use the app depending on the day or the moment.

Toys like these get used in lots of creative ways. A person with a clitoris might wear this kind of vibe while getting ready for a date night and control it themselves to "warm up" while still at home, then hand control to a partner as they head out together. Others rely on them as a way to stay connected while one partner is deployed or traveling for work. Some apps have built-in video and chat features, and some pairs of toys can also be synced. For example, one partner could be wearing a penis sleeve, and the other, a vaginal vibrator. Moving the penis sleeve causes the vibrator to rotate, and moving the vibrator causes the sleeve to squeeze.

Another less common variation is for an app-controlled vibrator or other toy to be worn to a dinner party, company function, or some other space where orgasms generally aren't expected, for the purpose of teasing or stimulating the partner. This does happen, though, perhaps more in fantasy than reality. These days, the idea of people secretly having orgasms in public places—the bar, the gym, while skateboarding in the park—is even its own porn genre. (Is there anything that *isn't* a porn genre?)

Being "Controlled" by a Partner

ALTHOUGH THE LANGUAGE of partner play with app-based toys is about "control," let's be clear: all healthy partnered sex is built on consent, even when the word *control* is part of the game. Controlling a partner or using a toy to stimulate them *without* consent is intimate partner violence and/or sexual violence, even if you never laid a hand on them or aren't even in the same state. The key to knowing it's legit is that the person whose body is being stimulated or "controlled" *chooses* to give that control to a partner, and has the power to end the game at any time by taking the toy out/off their body, or just communicating they need a break.

If app-controlled partnered sex experiences sound easier in theory than in practice, they can be. Experiences among our survey respondents were mixed.

Using an app-based sex toy with my partner was challenging at first because of the learning curve. Once we figured out the easiest rhythm, then app-based toys became our favorite for couple sex.

I struggle already with power dynamics, so I didn't like giving him that power.

It was more funny than anything. I don't think we were taking it too seriously.

I did this long ago, before there were toys built for it. A friend I fooled around with in high school just slid her phone into her panties on vibrate and I kept texting. I like to think I was ahead of my time.

Favorite Toy?

WE ASKED OUR vagina-owning survey respondents whether they had a toy they particularly like. Here are a few of the replies:

I like using a double-sided dildo in a harness. I love being able to stimulate my G-spot while also penetrating my partner.

A vibrator that's shaped like a stick, about five inches long. I like the consistency of the vibrations, like I don't get tired from my hand. I can also be specific with it because it's like a pencil. It's helped me realize specific parts that feel good to me.

I'm not proud to say this, but an Oral B battery-operated toothbrush without the brush head. Specific and amazing.

Regardless of how they're used, app-based toys are here to stay. The future holds a head-spinning (clit-spinning?) array of new options, including an expansion from toys that merely vibrate to full-on virtual reality sex experiences.

Trans Toys

PEOPLE OF ALL genders enjoy sex toys. If you've got a body part that likes a particular kind of sensation, there's a toy out there that will provide that. But despite the universal appeal, many toys are heavily gendered in their marketing. Sex toys are often pink with "pearls" or steely and rugged. Their packaging may suggest that only someone who identifies as a woman would enjoy using a certain toy when in fact anyone with a clitoris might find it delightful.

Thankfully, new companies like Hot Octopus, Cute Little Fuckers, and Perfect Fit Brand are making and marketing toys in an intentionally gender-expansive way. Avant sells dildos and other toys in the colors of the transgender, genderqueer, and asexual flags. Cute Little Fuckers describes their toys as "cute, shame-free, gender-inclusive, vibrating sex toys shaped like adorable monsters." Created by a gender-fluid and disabled engineer, each toy has its own backstory (and pronouns!), and some are designed to cover the genitals as they stimulate, which can be useful for folks who combat dysphoria by avoiding seeing or touching their genitals.

I don't have bottom dysphoria in the sense I want surgery; I'm totally fine with a vulva. I just can't touch myself with my hand. I usually use my vibrator or fingers over my underwear.

At the same time, sex toy companies are realizing there's a market—not just among trans people!—for toys whose packaging and design leave more room for possibility. A growing number of toys have sensual curves and colors that aren't gendered, recognizing that people of all genders might enjoy them. As the number of great options grows, the bigger challenge is choosing which one(s) you want in your bedside drawer!

I let my partner shop for toys for me because so many sex shops and toys are gendered and it feels really gross to shop in that kind of environment. But besides the marketing, toys aren't gendered and you shouldn't let their reputation scare you off.

Do Vibrator Lovers Still Want Partners?

AT ONE SPEAKING engagement, we could hear a couple of men in the audience grumbling as some women talked enthusiastically about how much they loved using vibrators. Finally, one guy raised his hand. "If girls are so into vibrators," he asked, sounding a little more miffed than he probably intended, "what do they need us for?"

We put the question to the people with a vulva who answered our survey: "If you can have an orgasm from a toy, do you still want to or enjoy having sex with a partner? Why or why not?" Here's what they had to say:

Oh, please. That's like saying if I could have a metal robot cat instead of a real one, I would want it instead. One purrs and is fluffy, soft, and warm, and the other is battery-powered.

Fret not, partners! Think of it this way: When we're using our vibrator, it's likely that we're thinking of you. When we're with you, do you really think we're fantasizing about being with our vibrator? Doubt it.

A plastic sex toy could never replace the warmth and feeling of my husband's hands, lips, and breath moving over my body. A sex toy might be a good thing to help stimulate a feeling or to appease a physical longing when he isn't around, but it in no way compares to the real thing.

Guys can have an orgasm any time they want by masturbating. I just find it quicker to use a vibrator. I'm a busy woman. I still enjoy sex with my boyfriend, and I usually prefer it. It's more intimate, more involved, multiple areas are stimulated, and after I masturbate I can't snuggle my vibrator.

Who wants a rubber fakey instead of human contact?! A vibrator doesn't involve another person's touch, or the excitement of not always knowing what comes next. Plus, you have to do all the work yourself.

The conclusion of the hundreds of people who shared their thoughts was clear: just because something can produce an orgasm doesn't mean it meets all the needs a partner can.

Other Toys

VIBRATORS MAY BE the most popular bedroom toy, but there's a vast universe of adult playthings. A few of the other top sellers:

Dildos

Dildos, toys designed for vaginal and/or anal penetration, are popular among those who enjoy the sensation of having something inside them. Dildos generally don't vibrate, but as we discussed earlier, some vibrators are phallic shaped and can be used as dildos. While some dildos are shaped like a penis (sometimes with veins, scrotum, and all), others look more like rippling magic wands in colors like magenta and periwinkle, or are strikingly clear with confetti floating inside. Dildos can also be worn with a harness as a strap-on; for more on that, see page 235.

I like my glass dildo I bought last year. It is clear and pink and very beautiful. I use it for G-spot stimulation.

I love a good ole fashioned dildo and harness for partnered sex.

Simple dildos, or items used as dildos, work best for me because they allow me to experience penetration while I stimulate myself.

I like using a vibrator and dildo combination. Usually one or the other can help me get there, but I have to finish with my hand. Using both I don't need to use my hands.

Anyone choosing a dildo can select exactly the width and length they find most pleasurable for penetration, an option not usually available when scoping out potential penis-wielding mates. If you're nervous about penetration, experimenting with a dildo at your own pace can help you gain confidence and comfort. Partners of all genders (including ones who have a penis) can also wear a harness and "strap on" a dildo, freeing up their hands for other

Ancient Inventions: The Wheel, the Calendar, the Dildo

DILDOS AREN'T EXACTLY newfangled: Archaeologists have found thirty-thousand-year-old specimens, and they show up in cave paintings of the time too. Around 500 BCE, the Greek port of Miletus became famed for the leather and wooden dildos it manufactured, which were designed to be used with olive oil for lube.

pleasures. If you buy a dildo with a suction-cup base, you can have hours of fun figuring out the best flat surfaces for riding (hint: the bathtub wall works well). These also make great conversation pieces when stuck to refrigerators and filing cabinets (in your home office, please).

Sexy Strap-Ons

SOME COUPLES HAVE great fun using a strap-on, a dildo worn in a harness. They're particularly popular for people with a vulva to be able to penetrate a partner of any gender.

Harnesses come in leather, vinyl, and rubber, with different designs depending on whether you want a center strap running between your legs or not. Most strap-on harnesses are designed for pelvic thrusting, but some people prefer thigh harnesses. Some harness designs give the wearer more clitoral pressure than others; some even have a pouch where the wearer can insert an egg vibrator. You can strap on a dildo of any size or style as long as it has a base wide enough to keep it in the harness.

Strap-ons can be worn by anybody. They're commonly used by lesbian, bi, and queer people with a vulva whose partners enjoy penetration. They're also a key ingredient in pegging, which usually entails a person with a vagina anally penetrating a person with a penis (see page 333). Thigh harnesses are popular with folks for whom age or disability makes pelvic thrusting difficult, or those interested in including penetration in their partnered sex when erections aren't possible.

My girlfriend and I bought a blue silicone unrealistic six-inch dildo and a nylon fabric harness. The dildo's name is Ernie.

I love my cock: It's huge and camouflage colored. I use it with a leather harness. I got it shortly before I turned twenty. I wanted a cock that I could identify with, that would feel like an extension of my own body, not a toy.

Wearing a strap-on has been very empowering. Getting close to orgasming without any physical stimulus and just mental. So that's cool.

There are also "strapless strap-ons," a dildo with a "bulb" at one end. A penetrating partner with a vagina inserts the bulb into their own vagina, while using the dildo end to penetrate their partner.

Regardless of what style you choose, it usually takes a while to get good at wearing and using a strap-on. There's a reason that teenagers with a penis tend to be awkward at intercourse at first. And people with a live penis don't have to worry about adjusting straps just so, having their tool flop away from their pelvis, or not being able to feel where they're thrusting! Like all things, practice helps, and it doesn't have to be a perfect performance for both partners to have fun. The person wearing the strap-on may want to penetrate their partner with fingers first, and then gently insert the dildo. The person being penetrated is always in charge because the vagina or anus has nerve endings and the dildo doesn't.

Strap-ons definitely aren't a requirement; some find it easier to use a dildo by hand, or aren't interested in penetration at all. But couples who love them think they're a pretty sweet invention.

G-Spot Toys

Sex toys designed for G-spot play generally have a bit of a curve, an angle, or an added bulb or ridge to help reach that sensitive area on the front wall of the vagina. Because G-spots usually respond best to firmer pressure, these toys are often made of a somewhat harder, less flexible material. To reach your own G-spot, insert one of these toys so the curve points toward your belly.

Masturbation Sleeves for Penis-Owners

These toys, sometimes known as strokers or by the best-known brand, Fleshlight, are designed to enhance the experience of penis stimulation. They come in different styles, often designed to mimic the look and feel of a mouth, vagina, or anus. In our survey, we asked penis-owners their thoughts, and they gave mixed reviews:

> It wasn't my favorite. I bought a high-end one so that I didn't make poor decisions with my sex life. It definitely helped me avoid making toxic booty calls. But I don't think it was worth it. You have to keep something like that very clean and it's a pain.

> I think that different sensations on the penis are fun and some guys feel like they should never experience that because of how stigmatized it is, but I think that if they tried it out, they'd see it as a means to enhance their masturbation.

Then, there's the DIY solution:

> As a kid I made a thing out of bubble wrap I filled with moisturizer and tucked under a pillow. It was awesome.

Butt Plugs, Prostate Stimulators, and Anal Toys

Back door toys have plenty of fans. Learn more about them in Chapter 11.

Toys as Tools for Mobility Issues

Sex toys can also expand the realm of possibility for people for whom sex can be physically challenging whether that's due to age, disability, or some other reason. If your hands have trouble with small manipulations like touching your clitoris, a toy can do the work. (It helps if it has big buttons or other easy-to-manipulate controls.) A dildo that can be moved by hand or strapped to a thigh or arm might be easier for some penis-owners than thrusting with a penis. Specialty pillows and wedges designed to make sex more comfortable can provide support where it's needed—and a stack of pillows or a rolled-up blanket can make a very suitable alternative for those on a budget. For books, websites, and social media accounts to explore these options in more depth, check out www.iloveorgasms book.com.

Keep 'Em Clean

SEX TOYS SHOULD be cleaned after each use. Putting a condom or plastic wrap on your sex toy makes it easy: just throw away the covering and put on a fresh one next time you're going to use it. If your friend wants to take your vibrator for a spin, make sure they condomize it too. If your toy isn't the right shape for a condom, or you opt not to use one, read the manufacturer's instructions to find out how to clean it, or check out websites on how to clean sex toys. Most materials can be washed with soap and water, or soaked or wiped down with a bleach solution (10 percent bleach, 90 percent water). Silicone toys that don't use batteries can be boiled or run through a dishwasher. Just don't forget to empty the dishwasher before your mom comes over, in case she gets inspired to help out!

Piercings

DO NIPPLE AND genital piercings improve orgasms? The answer depends on the person's body, the kind of piercing, and the type of jewelry worn after being pierced. Unfortunately, there's no way to know in advance whether you'll love the sensation or be eager to get the metal out of your pants.

While people often use shorthand like *clit piercing* and *penis piercing*, and there are plenty of jokes about the famed Prince Albert piercing, in reality there are literally dozens of basic types of genital piercings, plus more creative variations. If you're considering adding some body jewelry to your nipples or down below, you'll want to do your research and choose carefully. You'll also need to work with a knowledgeable piercer to be sure the type you've selected will work with your anatomy.

For all these kinds of piercings, some people find they enjoy the sensations of rubbing or tugging against the metal jewelry during masturbation or partnered sex, and some find the pierced body part becomes more sensitive (at least partly because they're more aware of it). For people with a clitoris, vertical clitoral hood, triangle, and Christina piercings (at the top of where the outer lips join together) seem to be the most likely to increase orgasm-related sensations because they can add pressure along the shaft of the clitoris, the area most people with a clit find most responsive. For people with a penis, apadravya or ampallang piercings (through the head of the penis) and genital beading are options said to be most likely to boost pleasure for the penis-owner's partner. Penis piercings may require a change in technique for how you put on a condom, and some kinds can increase the risk of condom breakage.

> *My labia piercing is fun because it reminds partners to play with my labia, which I really like.*

> *I've experienced climax-like feelings when just rubbing my pierced clit on my (female) partner's thigh.*

> *I had a mini-nipplegasm once by myself when I had nipple rings. It was definitely different from my normal rush—it was more of an all-over orgasm. I haven't been able to do it again.*

Piercing the clitoris itself is rare and considered potentially dangerous because of the risk of nerve damage. Most "clitoral piercings" actually run either above or below the glans.

Many people love their own or their partner's piercings for the aesthetics more than any enhancement in sexual pleasure. We've heard people say a sparkling ring changed their entire perception of their genitals, transforming parts they had found displeasing into art.

> *I feel like I'm sitting on a little silver secret.*

When I first got my nipples pierced, they became way more sensitive than before. I could get close to coming just from having my nipples played with (which I hadn't experienced before). Now, after five years, they don't feel any more sensitive than before they were pierced. I still love having my nipples played with, but the piercings are more for decoration than for sexual pleasure.

We *don't* recommend piercing as a way to solve orgasm difficulties. If piercing doesn't appeal to you, don't be talked into a piercing by a partner who promises

Flying High on the Nimbus

MATTEL, A TOYMAKER most famous for Barbie dolls and Fisher Price, isn't generally a player in the vibrator market. But when the Harry Potter craze was first heating up, Mattel designed a toy Nimbus 2000, a version of the flying broomstick that young wizard Harry rode while playing the sport quidditch. In addition to making "magical swooshing sounds," the battery-operated broomstick vibrated. What were kids supposed to do if they wanted to be just like young Harry? Turn the broom on, put it between their legs, and ride it!

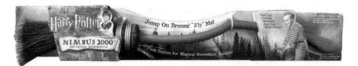

The toy got rave reviews on Amazon from parents astonished at how much time their adolescent daughters spent with it in their bedrooms ("I kind of wondered if she was too old for it, but she seems to LOVE it!"). Some moms reported riding the broom themselves on "a very magical journey." As the collection of ecstatic reviews grew, Mattel's higher-ups finally got in on the joke—and took the electronic broom off the market.

it'll change your sex life—there are no guarantees, and the unpierced can have perfectly mind-blowing sex lives. Given that you can't count on a piercing to add zing to your sex life, proceed with piercing only if you know you'll like the look.

I had my nipples and clitoral hood pierced. I was surprised that they didn't significantly change the way I experienced sexual pleasure. I ended up removing them because I noticed they made my partner less comfortable and less likely to contact those areas.

My vertical hood piercing gets in the way. I find that I have to take it out a lot during sex in order to get adequate clitoral stimulation.

Neither of my piercings enhance sensation that much, but they make me feel sexier. When my partner enjoys them, it relaxes me more and makes me get more into the mood.

Piercing carries real risks of infection and disease transmission, which can be particularly nasty when it's your nipple or genitals at stake. If you decide to get pierced, choose your piercer carefully. Visit the shop first, and check the piercer's credentials—safepiercing.org lists members of the Association of Professional Piercers. Ask about their safety and hygiene practices, and how many piercings they've done of the kind you want. You can set up a consultation appointment to get more information and let the piercer examine you to see whether your anatomy is compatible with the kind of piercing you want (not all kinds are compatible with all bodies) before you do the deed.

Concerned about the pain? That's also hard to predict: The same piercing can make one person almost pass out from the pain and can be just as easy as having one's ears pierced for another. As with ear piercing, those who are happy with their piercings typically say the short-lived pain was well worth it.

Toy and Piercing Tips for Partners

○ Be open to the idea that toys may enhance your shared sex life. Don't be threatened by a piece of plastic. Remember that even those who have great orgasms with vibrators crave the human connection of a partner—and frequently say that combining the two is the loveliest of all.

○ It can be easier to feel your partner's reactions when you're using your own fingers, tongue, or penis. When touching with a toy, be extra-attentive to your partner's reactions and facial expressions to be sure you've got the right angle or the right amount of pressure.

○ Don't pressure a partner to use a sex toy. It's great to be supportive of toy use or even to go shopping for a toy together, but remember that not every person is into sex toys. It's like having your parents pressure you to play soccer if playing trombone is really your thing. If *you* like toys, maybe it's time to do a little shopping for yourself!

○ Along the same lines, don't pressure your partner to get pierced if they're not into it. The risk, potential pain, and body modification aspects of piercing need to be freely chosen.

8

Come with Me
The Joys and Challenges of Partnered Sex

When most people think about orgasms, the image in their mind is partnered sex. And indeed, there's something that can be delightful and powerful about pleasure sparked by someone else's touch, and by sexual acts that require another person. A partner adds unpredictability to exactly how a given sexual interlude will go, transforming a solo only you control into an improvisational dance. Partners can do sexual things and reach sexual places that most of us can't do or reach ourselves. (Have you heard the classic joke: Why do dogs lick themselves? Because they can.) And of course, being with a partner often, though certainly not always, adds a level of emotional connection, meaning, and sometimes even (gasp!) love.

Getting Real About Porn

ONE OF THE challenges of partnered sex is that there's no simple, perfect way to learn how to do it, or how to do it well. So many things people do—cook meals, drive cars, clean toilets, resolve arguments—we first learned by watching our

Two by Two: Not for Everyone

IN OUR COUPLE-CENTRIC culture, it's easy to assume that being part of a couple is everyone's ultimate goal. While being part of a pair is a popular relationship choice, it's certainly not everyone's cup of tea. Some people prefer to have more partners, while others find solo singlehood to be their ideal. Asexual and aromantic people might want to be in a relationship, or might not.

I'm demisexual, so being with a partner and having sex with someone has never been a huge priority for me.

As I am on the asexual spectrum, I have little need for partnered sex. Partnered sex in general is more of an effort than enjoyment for me.

We explore asexuality more in Chapter 9.

Polyamory, meaning "many loves," is honest, ethical nonmonogamy, and can take many forms: an open relationship with one primary and the possibility of secondary partners, a triad with three equal and committed partners, a "vee" where two people are involved with the same partner but not with each other, and many more. Throughout this book when we write about partners, we do not assume that everyone has or wants only one!

parents or caregivers do the same activity. That's not the case with sex: the very thought makes most people shudder.

The sex ed taught to teens in schools is typically limited to the reproductive system and avoiding STIs and unplanned pregnancy; often not much relevant or useful information is provided to help you figure out what naked humans actually *do* in bed together, and how to make it feel good. "How to Help Someone Have an Orgasm" is definitely not in the curriculum. That leaves pornography, the only way that most people get to see other people have sex before having it themselves. There are massive generational differences here: Whereas older generations may remember swiping an old copy of *Playboy* and studying its pages furtively, today's middle schoolers can access literally millions of porn videos anytime they like, using the phone in their pocket that was conveniently provided by their parents. On average, kids today see porn for the first time at age eleven (sometimes on purpose, sometimes by accident). Porn is filling the gap, (poorly) answering common sex questions and satisfying curiosity. In our survey, 98 percent of cisgender men, 94 percent of transgender and nonbinary people, and 91 percent of cisgender women said they'd watched porn. And when we asked our survey respondents the different places they've learned about sex, 70 percent said porn was one of those. Only "friends," at 79 percent, ranked higher as a more common source of information.

Now, porn can be incredibly arousing. For some people it provides great entertainment for a Saturday night. And Sunday afternoon. And Monday during lunch break. If you want to have sex but have trouble getting turned on, porn might help. But porn also deserves the heaping serving of critique and criticism it receives; we'll be exploring this a bit more in this chapter. In the end, regardless of your opinion about its politics, morality, or arousal potential, porn is now part of most people's experience of learning about sex. Yet, as educational sources go, it leaves people wildly misinformed about the subject.

If some aliens were preparing a visit to Earth and decided they'd brush up on Earthling sex by watching the top videos on this planet's most popular porn sites, they'd probably conclude something along these lines:

1. Human bodies are mostly hairless (except for the hair on people's head).
2. Conventional beauty is a prerequisite for having sex. Only able-bodied people with a thin, toned body have it. Perky breasts and implants are the norm. No one has tummy rolls. Nearly all sex is had by people under age twenty-five unless one of them is a stepparent.
3. Sex is a performance. It needs to look good for the camera.
4. White people having sex with each other is the norm. When other races are involved, it's a unique category.

5. Talking is unnecessary. Consent never needs to be given or discussed.
6. Acts of physical and verbal aggression are commonplace.
7. Human penises are huge. And constantly hard.
8. People with a vulva get aroused with barely a touch and can quickly be in ecstasy no matter what the activity.
9. What sex is all about is a penis penetrating various orifices (mouth, anus, vagina).
10. Anyone on the receiving end of this penetration moans loudly in orgasmic ecstasy.
11. Once inside an orifice, the penis's job is to pound away, jackhammer style. The faster the better.
12. When the penis ejaculates, usually in the most dramatic way possible, the sex is over. Its owner's orgasm is the one that matters.

We cringe to imagine the scene if these aliens ever found themselves alone with consenting humans.

But that's exactly the challenge: just as aliens would be outsiders learning about human sex, almost all of us grow up as "outsiders" when it comes to learning how to have sex. And given how young most people are when they first encounter porn, it's not uncommon for people to have spent five to ten years having their mind filled with images of what sex supposedly looks like before they experience the real thing—and all too often try to replicate what they've been seeing.

We asked our survey respondents if there was anything they had to "unlearn" after watching porn. Here's a tiny snippet of the laundry list of things people mentioned:

You don't have to make porn noises. I think I've had to relearn what noises come out of me naturally.

Men rarely ever go near the clit, or if they do, they are aggressive with it.

Porn taught me that men are just animal-like sexual creatures, but they're more than that. When a male partner would simply need emotional support or a

The Challenge of Porn Stereotypes

MAINSTREAM PORN TENDS to perpetuate damaging stereotypes about people of color and lesbian, gay, and bisexual people while often erasing the existence of transgender and nonbinary folks. When there is trans representation, it is usually deeply fetishizing, rooted in shock value, and rather dehumanizing. Trans women are often used in scenes where a cis man is being humiliated and/or "emasculated" by her. Trans men are often misgendered or addressed in derogatory ways. And nonbinary people are...well, mainstream porn hasn't quite nailed down exactly how to fetishize nonbinary people yet.

Despite all that, it's also true that porn is the first time a lot of people see or learn about trans people. Maybe says: "I have suspicions about the effects that has on cis people's ideas of trans communities, but I also know that many trans people first discovered a connection to their gender while watching porn. Seeing a body that may look more like yours in sexual scenarios can be clarifying, even if the interactions being presented might be problematic. Obviously it's not the case for everyone, but there are trans and nonbinary people who first explored their gender after seeing themselves in porn."

It *is* possible to find ethical porn that's actually made for and by trans and nonbinary people outside the cis gaze, as well as porn made by and for cis women and/or lesbian, gay, or bisexual people.

shoulder to cry on, I would initially be confused, like, "You aren't tryna just make out?" Ultimately porn dehumanized men to me.

I actually had difficulty finding porn that spoke to what I wanted to see: a loving, consensual, long-term, intimate relationship focused on taking the time that both partners need to become aroused and ready for sexual activity.

It's okay to laugh and joke and be goofy during sex. You don't need to become a sex robot.

Many people specifically mentioned the violence and aggression that's the norm in much conventional porn, and the fact that it always runs the same direction, with people with a penis being aggressive toward people with a vagina.

Most women don't like to be slapped around and treated like crap in sex.

Porn shows men constantly demeaning women, so we're taught that that's what we should tolerate during sex. It teaches people that women are only objects of lust, never deserving of love, respect, or admiration.

Learning About Sex from Porn Is Like...

IN AN IMPASSIONED speech, actress Jameela Jamil said that in the absence of sex education about pleasure, porn becomes the substitute teacher for kids growing up today: "Learning to have sex from porn is like learning how to drive from *The Fast and the Furious*. A bloody horrendous idea." We think it's an excellent analogy.

Dorian has told bookworm middle schoolers that learning about sex from porn is like watching the movie before reading the book. The outline of the story may be there, but most of the best details are missing (and you'd have no idea about all the good stuff that's missing if you watch the movie first).

One of our survey respondents commented that porn is like pro wrestling; real sex is like regular wrestling.

What's your favorite "learning about sex from porn is like..." metaphor?

Do You and Porn Need to See Less of Each Other?

AUDIENCE MEMBERS SOMETIMES ask us our opinion of the NoFap movement, whose adherents choose to abstain from masturbation and porn. In general, we don't see a need to deny yourself the pleasure of masturbation, particularly over the long term. But porn can be a different story. If you're finding that after watching tons of porn—with its "horny stepsisters," enhanced body parts, and loud, fake orgasms—the sight of one normal, naked human in your bed is practically disappointing, then perhaps it is time to go on a self-imposed cold-turkey porn hiatus.

After watching porn, partner sex became different to me. Unless my girlfriend became the porn image, my penis stopped responding and I got turned off. Fantasies of the porn chicks dominated my head.

If you find that porn is interfering with your ability to enjoy your *real* sex life, you might consider a similar "trial separation." To do so, set a number of months (or weeks, or at least a number of days) for which you'll allow yourself no porn access at all. Then, pay attention to how it affects your thoughts and reactions to real partners, and decide at the end of that time what role you want porn to play in your life. Those who've tried it tell us they've been pleased with the results!

Fortunately, over time, it *is* possible to unlearn the messed-up messages porn sends. It's easy enough, after some reflection, to conclude that what works in porn often doesn't work in real life. The challenge is to figure out what *does* work with real, live human beings. Unlike the acrobatic, emotionless pseudo-sex in porn, this book is about the real thing. If you haven't already checked out these sections that definitely relate to partnered sex, we recommend you read up on:

○ The clitoris (see Chapter 1)
○ The G-spot (see Chapter 6)
○ Oral sex (see Chapter 4)
○ Penetration (see Chapter 5)
○ Helping a partner who's never (yet) had an orgasm (see Chapter 2)

The Orgasm Gap

STUDY AFTER STUDY documents a significant gender-based orgasm gap in hookups and relationships between cisgender men and women. Actually, it's more like an orgasm chasm. One study found that 91 percent of men said they'd had an orgasm the most recent time they'd had sex while 64 percent of the women said they had come. In another study, 95 percent of heterosexual women said their partner has an orgasm most or every time they have sex, but only 57 percent said the same was true for themselves. The situation is even starker in college hookups: 55 percent of men say they usually have orgasms during first-time hookups compared with 4 to 11 percent of women. Perhaps you won't be surprised to learn that lesbians have orgasms at about the same rate as straight men.

Interestingly, the orgasm gap isn't the same everywhere around the world. The orgasm gap in the US, Canada, Australia, Russia, Germany, Poland, the UK, Greece, and Thailand is up to twice as large as the gap in Singapore, China, Mexico, India, Spain, and Nigeria. The difference isn't baked into the vagina—clearly there are differences in how people are behaving sexually in these different cultures around the globe.

What's going on here? It's complicated. The biggest source of the problem is the belief that vaginal intercourse is expected in all, or at least most, sexual encounters. As you learned in Chapter 5, penis-in-vagina sex works great for leading to orgasms for penis-owners but is stunningly ineffective at helping vagina-owners find their O. Dr. Laurie Mintz puts it starkly in *Becoming Cliterate*, "Intercourse is the way men reach orgasm."

In the context of heterosexual college hookups, orgasms for cis women too often simply aren't on the agenda—it's nice if they happen, but neither partner generally expects it. But orgasms for cis guys are simply part of the script. Male pleasure is expected in hookups, much the way it is in conventional porn.

The fact that it takes longer for a person with a vagina to have an orgasm during partnered sex is a piece of the equation. (During masturbation, there's no difference in how long it takes.) Sometimes, couples just want a quickie. Or it's late and they're tired. It's easier to fit in a quick orgasm for a partner with a penis if it's a lunch break tryst or a few minutes before you both fall asleep.

The last piece of this puzzle is the way heterosexual cisgender women themselves are more likely than heterosexual cisgender men to say that they can enjoy sex without having had an orgasm. If at least some of the time, straight women say they're perfectly happy experiencing pleasure, and don't need an orgasm, that explains at least one slice of this gap.

Still, anyone who cares about fairness should be troubled by the persistent gap. The good news for straight people is that if you're reading this book, you're already well on your way to being better informed than most, equipped with a myriad of tools and strategies to shrink any gap in your own relationships. And the good news for LGBTQ people is that while individuals may, of course, have their own challenges, often there's no gap to worry about.

Seven Lucky Tips on Pleasing Your Partner

WE'VE TALKED TO thousands of people with a vulva about what makes a great partner, and what a partner can do to increase the odds of an orgasm. Besides the tips that appear elsewhere in the book, here's the best of our audience members' and survey takers' collective wisdom.

1. A great partner masters the art of foreplay. Many people think of "foreplay" as all the touching, kissing, stroking, caressing, nibbling, licking, whispering, and grinding that happens before penetration. But, of course, penetration is only one option on the sexual menu, and doesn't need to happen every time or at all. We believe foreplay *is* sex—many people of all genders find foreplay is the best, sexiest part of all. Calling it foreplay suggests that it's the opening act, the musician you listen to politely before the headliner (penetration) starts. Countless sexually experienced people have told us that some of the most thrilling, turned-on sex of their lives was as a teenager making out (foreplay!), months or years before they ever had intercourse. Foreplay can also be teasing through text messages; planning hot dates with each other and talking about what will happen; lying down naked and caressing each other; giving each other sexy eyes and flirting with no intention to have sex right away; and so much more.

No Wonder Lions Have That Look in Their Eyes

ACCORDING TO THE book *Biological Exuberance* by Bruce Bagernihl, a female lion "may mate as often as four times an hour when she is in heat over a continuous period of three days and nights (without sleeping), and sometimes with up to five different males."

Some scientists believe humans with a vagina need foreplay because they don't go into "heat" like most other mammals. Mammals with heat cycles are only sexually active certain times of the month (or year), but humans are lucky to be able to be aroused any day of the month. Foreplay is what gets the blood flowing.

Whether penetration is in the cards or not for a given sexual interlude, good foreplay boosts the chance your vagina-having partner will have an orgasm because usually that's what sends their arousal level sailing up, up, up. Orgasms take place only at the highest arousal levels—and foreplay is what moves the body and mind up the path.

2. A great partner asks (and listens). Many people imagine (incorrectly) that a great partner is so confident that they know exactly what to do to drive their partner wild. They also imagine (incorrectly) that if you're *not* sure, you should pretend you are, by never, ever asking for directions.

In fact, many of the world's best sex partners check in with their partners, ask questions, request feedback, and try out techniques many times, in many ways. This issue of asking—and listening to verbal and nonverbal cues—is just as relevant for a person who's never had sex as for one who's slept with a hundred

The Value of Slowing Down

IN OUR EXPERIENCE, it's almost unheard of for a person with a vagina to complain about a partner who spends too much time on foreplay. The reverse problem, partners who are in too much of a rush, comes up all the time as a source of frustration. If your partner has a vulva and you're not sure, err on the side of more foreplay than less foreplay.

My body is very sensitive and men tend to think they can take things so much faster than my body wants to go. My most amazing orgasms result from a very slow buildup that finally becomes completely overwhelming.

Help get me really aroused before you even think about touching my vulva. Wait until I crave that stimulation so much I feel as though I'm going to explode without it.

partners. And it's true for people of all genders—asking and listening isn't the job of only one partner or one gender.

For that matter, any attentive partner who has slept with more than one other person quickly realizes that what people like in bed, and how they respond sexually, varies so tremendously that it's not safe to assume that a new partner likes to be touched (or licked or penetrated) the same way the old one did. So, asking questions and checking in are not, as some fear, a sign of sexual cluelessness; to many vagina-owners, they're a sign of a partner who knows what it takes truly to give pleasure. As a bonus, all that checking in is a way of ensuring ongoing consent.

My last partner was the best. He asked me what I wanted, made it no secret that he enjoyed making me feel good, looked at my genitals, explored all my parts, took his time. He would keep things fresh by mixing up techniques.

Listening is probably the most important thing a partner can do. Someone who listens to what I like is the best at helping me have an orgasm.

Despite the mythology about a partner who just knows what to do (or thinks they do), most vulva-owners prefer a partner who communicates and asks questions. People with a vulva appreciate when a partner checks in as they move to start some new thing (and respect the answer). They give extra points to one who says, "I love feedback—tell me how I can make this even better for you." They adore a significant other who tries out a few different techniques (flicking their nipples with their tongue versus sucking on them versus gently biting them; a few different depths and angles of penetration; etc.) and asks which they most enjoy.

Communication during sex definitely does *not* have to mean long, clinical conversations. Lots of communication happens nonverbally, with moans and sighs, breathing that picks up, one partner moving another partner's hand to where they

Secrets of the Optometrists

HERE'S A TRICK to help you figure out what your partner likes. It's a technique with an unlikely source: the eye doctor. It's not actually all that surprising if you think about it: Eye doctors excel at figuring out what each stranger likes, what works best for their body. After you put aside all that med school technological stuff, they use a very simple technique: "A or B? B or C? C or D?"

Eye doctors give their patients simple options. Lots of options, two at a time. They ask you to choose, and they pay close attention to your answer.

How does this work sexually? You try two different ways of doing the same thing and ask, "Do you like it better when I touch this way, or this way? What about this way?" You can compare anything under the sun: Gentle bites versus kisses on the shoulder. A clit that's more responsive on the right versus the left. A left-handed versus a right-handed hand job. Different speeds, angles, or depths of thrusting. A more direct or less direct vibrator placement.

You don't need to use too many words. And definitely don't offer too many choices at once; two or three is ideal. Get your answer, do that for a while, then consider comparing that to something new.

You have what it takes to create a finely tuned map of your partner's most sensitive spots and favorite ways to be touched. Just channel your inner optometrist.

want that hand to be. But a certain degree of verbal communication is key too. Quiet appreciations can be super hot and help you both appreciate the moment. Complimenting how a partner smells or tastes, or the way their body feels against yours, is lovely. A low, sultry "Is this okay?" as one person's finger moves into their partner's underwear, or as a head arrives between the other's thighs, can be answered with an appreciative, "Mmm-hmm." Not only does this *not* break the mood, it enhances it, knowing that your partner actually cares. And if someone's answer is "Not yet" or "Let's try this first," a great partner wants to know that—and is ready to respect limits and pace each step of the way.

Ease your way down my pants. The longer you take to get there the better. I feel the sexiest and most turned on the more I'm caressed. It's all about desire. I need to feel comfortable, so always ask if it's okay. And then take your time.

3. A great partner knows what to do with a clitoris. First, know where to find it. Second, don't rush for the clit too early. Some penis-owners would be thrilled if their partner started rubbing their penis within the first minute of making out. Most clitoris-owners don't want the same kind of immediate attention to their clit. For clitoral touching to feel good, most people need to be aroused already. (The question of how early in a sexual interlude a partner would enjoy a hand between their legs is a fun, and fascinating, conversation to have with a partner since people's preferences vary widely.)

My boyfriend asks me what I like and don't like, so I tell him and show him exactly how I want to be touched. His techniques I like best are when he uses lots of lube and massages my clitoris with his middle finger. He asks me how I want it, so I tell him faster, slower, harder, in circles.

Third, check in with your partner to find out how that person's clit likes to be touched, realizing that this likely changes as arousal climbs. Watching your partner masturbate (and being willing to let them do the same) can offer fantastic insights if you're both comfortable with the idea. And finally, remember that for most vulva-owners (though not all), clitoral stimulation is the primary route to orgasm. If one partner or the other doesn't spend some time making sure this gold nugget gets its share of attention, orgasms will probably be hard to come by.

One study found that if a partner spends at least twenty minutes doing clitoral stimulation—that could be caressing through clothes, gentle massage with fingers, oral sex, and so on—more than 90 percent will have an orgasm.

4. A great penis-owning partner knows the penis is merely one tool among many. Penises are a pretty remarkable invention, no question about it. Yet those who don't have one have been known to complain privately that many penis-owners' love of their favorite body part distracts them from the wonders of everything else they have to offer. It's up to each partner to prove they know how to use the whole toolbox. (For more on this, see page 251.)

Patience is unquestionably a trait to cultivate if you're working toward an I Orgasm merit badge. (If you're not clear on how long orgasms can take, see page 27).

5. A great partner masters the art of patience. One of the greatest gifts anyone can give their vulva-owning partner—especially one who worries that they're taking too long to have an orgasm—is to say honestly, "Let's keep doing this as long as it feels good to you. I'm not in a rush. I'm enjoying this too." You may have to offer repeated reassurance, especially if the activity in question is one that centers on a vagina-owning partner's pleasure!

Here's a common example: Lots of people with a vulva enjoy receiving oral sex. Lots of partners do, too, but don't spend enough time down there to have it lead to orgasm.

One solution: Test your sense of time against your phone or the bedside clock. In your head, privately come up with a minimum amount of time that you're going to perform oral sex; let's say thirty minutes. Sneak a peek at the time as you start, and then don't look at it again until you *think* thirty minutes has passed. When you sneak your second peek, you may be surprised at how little time has actually passed. It's easy to lose track of time in bed! So, get back to it!

I want to feel that however long it takes me to reach orgasm is fine, and that it's okay if I want to have more than one, and that if I need to have them after your orgasm that you won't roll over and neglect me. I won't want to get very aroused if I don't think you'll stick around through it.

It's a lot easier to be patient if you're comfortable. For anything you plan to do for a while, it helps to be in a position that isn't going to strain your neck or make your arm fall asleep. And don't be afraid to tell your partner if you need to switch positions, grab a pillow, or change something slightly. You can make it clear that you're still all in and eager to continue as soon as adjustments are made.

6. A great partner knows that vulva-owners come first (at least some of the time). For different-sex couples, orgasm connoisseurs know that it often works better when the vagina-owning partner comes before the one with the penis. If the vulva-owner's pleasure is the first priority, the penis-owner is likely to stay awake and engaged for the whole process, right through to their own orgasm. Plus, given how arousal works for people with a vulva, there's a good chance the vulva-owner will be happy to continue until the penis-owner comes—maybe even going on to have another orgasm or two.

The fact that my boyfriend wanted me to orgasm before he did was so sweet. He had such determination to make me happy that it helped me.

My last boyfriend almost always was able to make me climax and probably was the best person I've ever had sex with. He was very giving and would almost always go down on me prior to us having intercourse. This would help in that I'd be wet enough for him to enter me without too much discomfort.

7. A great partner makes it clear they're enjoying themselves (if they are). We hear people of all genders say they prefer a partner who makes it easy to see and hear when they're enjoying themselves. Lots of us trained ourselves to be silent in our earliest sexual experiences, perhaps at home with the risk that parents might overhear or in a dorm where sound travels far too easily, and for some people that habit sticks. Once you're an adult having sex in a place where silence isn't required, remember that authentic moans, gasps, whimpers, and sighs of pleasure are often turn-ons for both partners. When things feel great, don't be afraid to use words and sounds to let your partner know!

I wish men would vocalize their own pleasure more. Knowing that my partner is enjoying the experience is perhaps the best part of a sexual encounter and allows me to get more aroused and more likely to reach orgasm.

Consent Without Awkwardness

[Content note: The first paragraph and the box Learning to Consent mention sexual violence.]

A truly excellent partner wants to have sex with someone who wants to have sex with them. But talking about consent with someone you're hoping to get it on with—or are already sleeping with—can feel intimidating. For many people, the fear is that if you ask, your partner might say no. But if you don't ask, maybe you can get away with it? That's bad form and unsexy—don't do it. By definition, sex without consent is sexual assault. Sexual assault can include any kind of unwanted touching of someone's breasts, butt, or genital areas, not just penetration, and doesn't need to involve force or physical violence.

So, to do it right, you and your partner actually have to communicate about what you're going to do before you do it. Even if checking in feels awkward, you still need to do it. Most people are charmed by a partner who asks, even awkwardly.

Learning to Consent

MAYBE SAYS: AS a survivor, I didn't understand consent for a very long time. When I was abused for multiple years as a teenager, I was unable to consent at all because I was underage. But my confusion continued into my early adulthood. I understood that one could say no, even though I didn't actually know how to go about saying it. What I didn't know at the time was that I could say yes. Because my first and only experience with sex was that it happened *to* me, it never occurred to me that it was something I could choose to invite. Years later, the first time a partner asked before touching me, I was so confused. It was my first time consenting to sex.

But it doesn't have to be super awkward. Our favorite tool for this situation is the phrase, "Is this okay?" To use it, you make it clear what you're interested in without quite doing the thing. Maybe you put your fingers on the button of your partner's jeans or their bra clasp, start to reach your hand under their underwear, or slide a finger in the direction of their anus. Then, you pause and say the magic words, "Is this okay?" We recommend your favorite quietly steamy voice. Pause and let your partner respond. A lack of response equals no. "I'm not sure" also equals no. Hesitation and reluctance: both no's. And if you get a no, you can softly kiss them (or some other type of expression of affection you know your partner is comfortable with) and say, "No problem," and then smoothly continue with what you were doing before. But you might get a yes—maybe even an enthusiastic one.

Of course, a single yes doesn't unlock the wonders of the sexual universe for the night ahead. You have to check in again each time you want to take things further or try something new. You can use even shorter phrases: "Okay?" "All right?" and "This good?" all fit the bill. Most important is that you're listening to and respecting the answers you get.

Which partner's job is it to get consent? Both—but especially whoever is suggesting a new activity, or beginning to take things to the next level. Too often, consent is discussed as a man's responsibility, but it's actually about behavior, not gender.

Discussing and negotiating consent plays out a little differently in longer-term relationships. While consent is essential in *all* relationships, long-term couples who have already negotiated consent in the past and established a set of "these are things we like to do sexually" may not need the same degree of checking in each and every time. But if one of them expresses hesitation or disinterest, even in something they've liked in the past, the same consent rules still kick in.

Maybe Says: Body Tours for Everyone

ASSUMPTIONS ABOUT EACH other's body affect everyone who has partnered sex. Many cisgender folks have had the experience of someone attempting to stimulate or pleasure their body but getting it wrong, perhaps because they assume that what will turn on a new partner is exactly what turned on the last partner. For nonbinary and transgender people, a partner's assumptions can misgender them or result in language or touch that doesn't feel affirming for them.

A wonderful technique I've learned is to give your partner a body tour. This can be a sexy and playful way for couples of any combination of gender identities (this means you, too, cis people!) to show your partner where you like being touched, tell them what you like your parts to be called, and more! And of course your partner can do the same for their body. You can start with naming what areas are okay or off-limits, or identifying parts of your body and what you like them to be called. This can happen before the encounter, outside the bedroom, or even over texts. It could mean turning all the lights off and describing a scene together. In this shared fantasy, each partner can describe their body to be exactly what they want it to be, and it can function how they desire. Feel out what works best for you and your partner, and see how much you can learn about each other by communicating about desire and pleasure.

> *I like to explain how things feel and what words I use to describe things and what feels comfortable. I also explain the correct way to touch my chest that feels comfortable. I don't want my chest to be grabbed, but I like when someone's hand is on my chest and playing with my nipple or touching my skin. I also explain the right way to touch me between my legs.*

> *I tend to do that outside the bedroom with clothes on because then I feel more like they're listening and I don't feel like I'm objectifying myself, nor am I trying to give a lecture while feeling very exposed.*

Body tours aren't useful only for navigating dysphoria. Sexual assault survivors have also found them helpful, as well as others who've had trauma affect their body in ways that their partners might need to be aware of. They can also be helpful for people who have medical issues that affect how they can use their body during sex.

I have PCOS [polycystic ovary syndrome], which can trigger periods of chronic pain. This typically means a pre-sex conversation about certain positions or methods that may cause pain at that time, even if it's not typically painful when I am not experiencing a flare-up.

When we asked about body tours on our survey, there were plenty of enthusiasts—and even more who said things like "Wow, no, but I love this idea and can't wait to try!"

Like many things, I try to imbue it with humor and levity. I think for me it makes it accessible and not awkward. I've had it not go well a few times and then I just simply see myself out of the situation.

The Power of Renaming Your Genitals

RECLAIMING YOUR BODY and the ways that you talk about it can also be really effective for trans and nonbinary people. Especially for people who have not had or do not want certain gender affirmation surgeries, the language they use to describe their body can be really important. We asked survey takers who hadn't had genital surgeries what words they use to describe their genitals. Some mentioned that they don't like to use language for their genitals at all, but many did have answers. At the risk of reinforcing the binary, we've listed them in categories based on sex assigned at birth.

People who were assigned male at birth:

bits	genitals
clit	girldick
clitty	penis
coochie	pussy
cunt	shenis
dick or cock	vagina
front parts	

People who were assigned female at birth:

bits	innie
bonus hole	junk
click (clit + dick)	lips
clit	mancave
cock	me
cockpit	parts
coochie	penis
cunt	pussy
delicate flower	stuff
dick	T-dick
front hole	vagina
genitals	yoni
hoo-hah	

Faking

AN ORGASM IS a beautiful thing. Most people would like to see more of them in their lifetime. But is seeing believing? A lot of folks start squirming uncomfortably in their seat when the issue of faking comes up. Depending on the study, research finds that between one-third and two-thirds of women have faked an orgasm at least once. Despite all those fake orgasms, only 20 percent of heterosexual men think their partners have ever faked. (That must be some pretty good acting!) You might be surprised to learn that penis-owners also fake orgasms: newer research found that a full 16 percent of their orgasms are also fake. We have not found data on this subject about trans and nonbinary people. You have questions on the subject? We've got answers.

First things first: *Is there any way to tell for sure whether a person with a vulva is faking or not?*

Some partners have heard that you can recognize a real orgasm by physical signs like a red flush on the face or neck, vaginal contractions, spasms or tremors throughout the body, curled toes, hard nipples, dilated pupils, elevated heart rate, or a quivering lower lip. Indeed, each of those things *can* be present when a person with a vulva has an orgasm—but they would more accurately be considered signs of arousal (or, in the case of hard nipples and dilated pupils, they could be an indicator that your bedroom is cold and dark). Many vulva-owners experience some combination of those physical effects when they're aroused—whether they have an orgasm or not. Nearly all can easily be faked.

But wait. How do people with a penis fake?

The faking itself is the easy part: Penis-owners can moan and shudder just as well as their vagina-toting counterparts. The lack of evidence of ejaculate creates an extra hurdle for penis-owners who didn't really come. But during vaginal or anal penetration, that's simple enough to fake since that ejaculate isn't readily visible anyway. They can always tie up and throw away an empty condom. Or they can claim that the (nonexistent) amount of ejaculate is very small because they'd masturbated earlier in the day. Most of the time, partners probably aren't paying such close attention.

But surely there must be some way to spot a fake?

There is: Through the use of a positron emission tomographic (PET) scanner. This useful device, which costs a mere $2 million, can measure the activity in your partner's cerebral cortex. But without a PET scanner, no, there's absolutely no way to accurately distinguish an orgasm from a talented acting job.

But here's the deal: Rather than agonizing over the authenticity of the orgasms, focus instead on the root cause of faking by not pressuring your partner to have an orgasm. Some partners couldn't care less about pleasure and orgasm. If you're reading this book, you're probably not one of them—you *do* want the person or people you sleep with to have a good time. But there's another kind of partner: the ones who care too much.

Some partners get it into their head that because of their lovemaking prowess, orgasm is a gift they bestow upon their vagina-having partners. They see it as a personal challenge to make their partner come. Whether it's spoken aloud or not, people quickly catch on to the fact that it would make their sweetie really happy if they had an orgasm. But, as we've discussed throughout this book, there are any number of reasons why they might not be able to have one, reasons that have nothing to do with the partner's lovemaking skills.

If a partner is trying really hard—with tongue, fingers, penis, or sex toy—to help a vulva-owner have an orgasm, and the person with the vulva suspects (or knows) it's just not going to happen, they may start to get nervous, tired, or sore. Those states make it even harder to come, and the orgasmic brass ring begins to slip out of reach.

I had a boyfriend who I had to fake it with for a long time. No matter how much I tried to help, he didn't want to listen to my advice, but he wouldn't stop until I supposedly "had one."

Being designated female at birth, I felt a lot of pressure to orgasm when I was with my first boyfriend, and felt like I had to fake orgasming or be extra loud and physically expressive to make him happy.

For some people with a vulva, faking provides an easy solution. The orgasm-obsessed partner thinks their partner had an orgasm, so they're happy. The orgasm faker is happy because the partner is happy. All is well and good—until the next time they're in bed together when the partner repeats the same techniques, thinking they worked last time, and the past faker is faced with the same dilemma. The cycle repeats itself until either the faker fesses up and the two of them have a heartfelt conversation about it, or they break up—possibly the opportunity to deliver the news: "Oh yeah, and one other thing: I've never had an orgasm with you! I was FAKING every time!" Those are words nobody ever wants to hear.

If that's the case, what's the use in trying?

Somebody smart once said, "Live for the journey, not the destination." Sex is about more than achieving orgasm. It's also about intimacy, love, the thrill of skin against skin, human connection. It is absolutely, genuinely possible to have a *great* time having sex, yet have no orgasm. Most people with a vulva, in particular, say that at least some of the time, they can be perfectly satisfied without coming.

> *If I tell you I don't think I can have an orgasm—and sometimes I can tell it just isn't going to happen—don't belabor the point. Enjoy yourself, come, and don't feel bummed that I didn't come, because I really DID enjoy being with you!*

Here's the bottom line of what vulva-owners want from their partners: Do things that focus on their pleasure, be really, really patient, and let go of the end goal of an orgasm. By "focus on their pleasure," they usually mean oral sex or gentle clit massage with your or their own fingers or a vibrator, not just penetration. By "really, really patient," they mean allow twenty to forty minutes or more if the person with the vagina is enjoying themselves and says they'd like to continue. Be happy if your partner is happy, whether or not there are fireworks in the end.

Faking Dos and Don'ts (for people who have faked or are tempted by it)

1. DO consider taking a no-faking pledge. Making a personal no-fake orgasms pledge is a promise to yourself that you're going to be a person who doesn't fake it. Ever. If you make this commitment, it pretty much guarantees there will be at least some sexual situations in your life when you don't have an orgasm, and your partner will know it. Get okay with that. Realize that in the long run, some orgasm-free sex episodes are far better than "training" your partner to repeat an ineffective technique on you and every future vulva-owner they sleep with. As one of our friends said, "Every faked orgasm moves humanity further from achieving a real one."

Are You on the Ceiling, or Inside Your Own Body?

ONE VERY COMMON barrier that can interfere with people's (especially vulva-owners') ability to experience pleasure is called "externalizing." It means that instead of experiencing the sensations in your body, you're watching yourself—and probably being your own meanest critic. Externalizing is something our brain learns to do because we're insecure, because porn teaches us that sex is a performance for *watching* rather than experiencing, because we can't turn off our negative body self-talk.

Because of our society and culture, the male gaze was so ingrained that during sex I was always only worried about how the man was perceiving me rather than my own experience.

Being aware of myself and how I look from the outside usually cuts me off from my own pleasure more than anything. It's best when I can stop focusing on how I look.

We wish human brains came with a Settings menu. Then, we'd just tell you to toggle the Externalizing switch to off, and that would be the end of that problem! Solving this isn't quite that easy. But when you catch yourself watching yourself during sex, take a breath, reenter the *inside* of your body, and remind yourself it's what you *feel* that matters right now, not how you look.

My first girlfriend faked it—quite poorly—and it had negative effects on our relationship. My last girlfriend never faked. We talked about my performance. When it wasn't good, I wanted to know so I could improve.

If your partner knows you're honest when you don't come, they can also begin to trust that when you do scream their name or grab onto their shoulders, that orgasm was for real. That kind of trust and honesty builds great relationships inside the bedroom and out.

You may have noticed that we said, "Consider." We used to recommend that everyone pledge not to fake. We still think that's sound advice. But we've become convinced that for a small percentage of people, there may be situations where faking is to your advantage. We read about a woman who loved sex of all kinds but well into her thirties had never had an orgasm. She experienced ecstatic pleasure, though, and very much enjoyed the sex she had. She was in a long-term relationship with a man who was orgasm obsessed, who just couldn't let it go and felt her lack of orgasms was hurting his own self-esteem. So, she started faking for his sake, and it solved what had been a major relationship problem. If you find yourself in a long-term relationship like this, and you're comfortable *never having an orgasm*, then go for it and fake. It's not your fault that your partner has lost sight that it's your *pleasure* that really matters. But be warned: once you start, it's extremely difficult to return to trying to have real orgasms.

The same may be true in a one-night stand–style hookup when things are starting to chafe and your partner seems intent on pumping away until you come. Maybe faking then is simply expeditious. But on the whole, it would be better if hookups trended toward more honesty too. (Suggesting a slower pace or a change of activity, adding more lube, or saying, "I don't think I'm going to come tonight, but it's fine for you to. This was really fun," would all be reasonable, more honest options for this situation.)

2. DO break the cycle if you've been faking. Your pseudo-gasms may not matter if it's a short-term fling or if you're about to end things anyway. But if this is a long-term love, or a new relationship you think has potential, you owe it to yourself to help your partner help you have real orgasms.

Obviously, if you like this person, you don't want to hurt their feelings. Let's say you've been faking orgasms after five minutes of oral sex, and you suspect you could come for real if the stimulation continued longer. Here's one approach that's only half honest but may do the trick to get you back on track without causing a major crisis: "Honey, I've been reading this book about orgasms. There was a section about how orgasms can feel, and how long it can take a lot of us to get there.

It got me wondering if I could have bigger orgasms if we did stuff for longer—sometimes it feels really, really good, but the more I read, the more I'm not sure whether I'm having orgasms all the time or not. Would you be up for trying some different things, or just going for longer, to see how it feels for me?"

If you have real orgasms sometimes but fake when you can tell it's not happening (so your partner *thinks* you come every time), try gradually cutting back on your faking. Sometimes, when you can tell an orgasm just isn't meant to be, don't fake—let your partner know you had a good time but you're not going to come tonight. Gently introduce the idea that sometimes you come and sometimes you don't, reassuring your partner that an orgasm isn't the only thing that determines whether you enjoyed yourself. (It takes some partners months or years of reassurances to become comfortable with the idea that many people with a vulva can enjoy sex whether or not they have an orgasm every time.) Intersperse real, fake, and nonorgasms, gradually providing fewer fakes and allowing sex without orgasm to happen from time to time. As your partner adjusts to the idea that you don't always come—and that you're okay with that—phase out your faking entirely.

3. DO be firm and honest if you're being pressured. If you get the sense your partner's pride hinges on whether you come, you may begin to dread what's ahead. Rather than just enjoying each other, the interlude has been transformed into a test of performance, your partner's and yours. When a partner tells you your orgasm is their goal or keeps asking whether you came, be kind but clear: "Sometimes, I have orgasms; sometimes, I don't. That's not really the point. I love being with you; it feels really good." Give them positive feedback for the things they're doing that you like ("I love how long you go down on me" or "You feel so good inside me"). If you have ideas for what could help you come, share them. In the end, be honest about how long you want the pleasuring to continue, and, if you're asked, whether you did or didn't have an orgasm. Your significant other may need to be reassured many times that you don't need to have an orgasm every time to consider it great sex and be totally satisfied—many people with a penis, in particular, can't imagine this could be true. Over time, your partner will come to respect your honesty and be less invested in your orgasm as the only sign that they did a good job. You may be rewarded with a more relaxed partner. Without the pressure, you might be able to breathe easier too—which, ironically, could lead to more orgasms.

Faking Dos and Don'ts (for partners)

1. DON'T announce, "I'm gonna make you come." That is, unless your goal is to receive a fake orgasm. A partner who hears words like these feels incredible pressure to make you happy. Their orgasm becomes something that's for *your* pleasure rather than their own. And if it's for your pleasure, they figure, they might as well put on a good (fake) show for you to enjoy.

2. DON'T ask, "Did you come?" As much as you might be tempted to inquire, keep your curiosity to yourself. It's too difficult to answer: If they say no, they'll worry you'll be disappointed. If they say yes, you'll have no way of knowing if they're lying or telling the truth. Also, if they did have an orgasm, they don't need a reminder that their real orgasms don't involve the artificial moans and screams one sees in movies and porn. The last thing your partner should have to worry about at the moment of their peak pleasure is whether they're being expressive enough to let you know they're having an orgasm! That said, after you've been together at least a few times, it's okay to say, "Sometimes it's hard for me to tell whether you have orgasms." Let them answer, and listen. Follow up with "Are there things I could do differently to help you?" Communicate with your words and reactions that you're okay if your partner has an orgasm or not, as long as you're doing what you can to make sure they're enjoying themselves.

3. DON'T fake orgasm yourself. This applies to people of all genders, including penis-owners. Given that penis-owners usually ejaculate when they orgasm, it's a bit harder to fake, but it's certainly not impossible:

> *If we're having intercourse for a second time in a short period of time, I usually keep going until she's had another orgasm, and then I fake an ejaculation. Yeah, it can be done with a bit of acting, as well as flexing the muscle down there. Women aren't the only ones who can fake it.*

The Golden Rule is apropos here: Do yourself and your partner a favor, and don't fake. If you both have a vulva, it's only fair that you both play by the same set of rules—or that you model how it's possible to be honest while still having fun and being appreciative of the pleasure your partner provides. If you have a penis, it's perfectly normal occasionally to lose your erection during sex, and partners need to understand that. There's no need to fake to cover up what happened. Penis-owners are not infallible machines, but human beings with body parts that have a mind of their own.

4. DO be wary of orgasms that are too good to be true. If you're a penis-owner whose vagina-having partner always has a simultaneous orgasm with you after two minutes of intercourse, know that while such a feat is physically possible, it's quite rare. Of course, don't make the mistake of accusing your partner of faking, lest you offend one of the few lucky vulva-owners on earth who can come that quickly and easily. But don't be lax about following all the other suggestions in this chapter, like providing ample opportunity to get off in other ways.

5. DO accept a faking confession graciously. If a partner ever admits to you that they faked an orgasm, stay calm and thank them for their honesty. This news can be frustrating to hear, but no one wants to be stuck having dishonest sex forever. Your partner just gave you the gift of truth. Now it's your turn to use this newfound knowledge as an opportunity to get back on track and figure out how to work together (it's both partners' responsibility) to achieve the real thing—or embrace that pleasure is the real goal, not orgasms.

Spicing It Up: A Game for People in Long-Term Relationships

HERE'S ANOTHER QUESTION that's all too common among those who've logged many hours together between the sheets: "My partner and I have good sex, but we always do basically the same things. How can we spice it up?" Figuring out how to shatter the monotony or expand your sexual horizons is one part of the challenge; the other is how to start the conversation.

Here's a creative, nonthreatening way to dip a toe (or some other body part) into the pool of possibilities. Do this when you both have some free time, like during a long walk, a long drive, or while lazing around together in bed.

Step one: Together, brainstorm sexual activities that you haven't done together (or haven't done much). You can write things down if you want to, but you don't have to. Think as broadly as you can, large and small, meek and wild. There are no wrong answers—just because you name an activity doesn't mean you want to do it. In fact, the game is more fun if you name things that don't interest you as well as things that do.

Step one, the shy version: If you or your partner are the kind who blush easily, each of you take your own piece of paper (or start a password-protected note app on your phone), and individually brainstorm as many sexual things as you can think of. Afterward, share your lists with each other.

Step two: As you brainstorm, for each activity that either of you names, you each say whether it's in your personal "Yes," "No," or "Maybe" category. "Yes" means it's something you'd like to try. "No" means you wouldn't do it under any circumstances. "Maybe" means you might be open to it if all the conditions were right, or willing to try it if your partner were excited about it. Here's a snippet of a sample conversation between two people:

Person #1: *How about toe-sucking. Would you want to try toe-sucking?*

Person #2: *Ewww!*

#1: *What if we washed our feet first and then tried it?*

#2: *It sounds weird—but I guess I'd be willing to try it if our feet were clean. Maybe.*

#1: *I'd say yes for me.*

#2: *Okay, let's see. . . . How about having sex outdoors?*

#1: *Like that night out at the lake? That was great! Yes, definitely.*

#2: *Okay, yes for me too. Let's do more of that.*

#1: *Ummm . . . spanking?*

#2: *No, I definitely don't like being spanked.*

#1: *I'm not really into that, either, so "no" for both of us.*

#2: *I thought of one! I always thought it would be fun to kiss for really long, just keep kissing and kissing and kissing and kissing.*

#1: *Uh, sure. I never really thought about it, but yeah, I'm willing to do that.*

#2: *What about tying each other up?*

#1: *I don't know, I don't like the idea of being tied up.*

#2: *How would you feel about tying me up? Like with neckties or something.*

#1: *(giggling) You'd want me to tie you up?*

#2: *I think it could be fun to try.*

#1: *Really? Okay, I'm fine tying you up—I just don't want to be tied up.*

#2: *Okay, so we both say yes to you tying me up, and you say no to me tying you up.*

#1: *All right, here's another one . . . [and the conversation continues]*

Step two, the shy version: Each of you take a new sheet of paper, or create a new three-column note. Label your three columns "Yes | Maybe | No." Categorize each of the sexual activities you and your partner brainstormed into one of the three categories. When you're both finished, share your papers with each other.

Step three (the same for regular and shy versions): Once you have a good list—or you're running out of time—review the activities that you both said yes to. There's your list to start with—have fun! You can also review the ones that got one "Yes" and one "Maybe." For the ones that got a "Maybe," talk about why each of you put it in the category you did, and under what conditions you'd be comfortable giving it a go. Keep in mind that no matter how long you've been together, consent is never something to take for granted. Particularly when you're venturing into new areas, be sure you're on the same page. Saying yes to something on paper doesn't mean you can't change your mind!

THE HIGH-TECH VERSION, suitable for shy people: We think there's both value and fun in the process of brainstorming, dreaming, giggling, and talking about potential sexual adventures. But there are also apps and websites that will facilitate the game for you (we'll list some on the book's website). They all operate similarly: you and your partner share a link that connects you to each other. Then, the app generates a list of possible activities, some milder, some bold and spicy. Each partner privately selects yes, no, or maybe for each item.

When you've both finished, the app compares your answers and displays for both of you *only the items to which you both said yes or maybe.* So, if you're a little embarrassed to admit you've always wanted to try watersports or fantasized about role-playing sexy nurse—well, your partner won't find out unless they, too, checked the box to say they're interested in the same thing.

FOR ADVANCED PLAY: Here's a twist for the daring. Follow the previous advice for the shy players, so you each end up with separate "Yes | Maybe | No" lists. (Or use the shared Yes and Maybe lists generated by your app.) Compare lists, taking a good look at what's in your partner's "Yes" category that you haven't done together, or haven't done much.

Then, set a "date night" and designate one of you as the Planner. The Planner makes all the arrangements for the night, which could include dinner at the other partner's favorite restaurant or other treats. Afterward, the Planner takes the lead with sex, focusing exclusively on activities that are in their partner's "Yes" category. The partner's job is simply to enjoy! Next time, switch roles, with the other person taking the lead.

In a long-term relationship, this is the kind of game you can repeat from time to time as the years go by. You may be surprised to learn that things commonly shift around: One person's "No" transforms into a "Maybe," and a "Yes" becomes a "No." As you explore together, you'll get new ideas, decide to return to things you did when your relationship was new that you've since drifted away from, perhaps feel more adventurous in one area and clearer that you don't enjoy something else. The goal is *not* to try to prove how kinky you can be, and it's definitely not to push people to do things that don't appeal to them; each person's "No" category must be respected. Really, it's just a fun way to have a conversation—hopefully one that leads you to some ideas that banish bedroom boredom.

For Trans Folks Navigating Partnered Sex

Communication

FOR TRANS AND nonbinary people, trying to embark on a sexual interaction without having a conversation first can result in your partner making loads of assumptions. If your partner has never had sex with a trans person before, they might presume they know how your body will look or respond. If they have had sex with a trans person before—the same thing could happen. Trans people, like all people, want and enjoy different things, and how pleasure works for any one of us can't be assumed.

Most of our survey participants who've had partnered sex have been out to at least some of those partners. Some of them commented on how they handled that.

In the past, I've had to correct partners about the specific words I use to describe my body (clit versus penis/cock, and how to refer to my chest, for example). I have to correct people about my identity a lot and make it clear that I'm nonbinary, and that no matter how I present or behave, that does not mean I identify with a binary gender.

I explain it as simply as possible: "Yes, I have breasts, yes, I am a man," and move on.

For one-night stands I don't usually take the time to educate them unless they're ignorant—in which case I usually cancel our plans anyway—but if I'm with someone with whom I'd like to develop a relationship, I take it upon myself to educate them slowly but surely. It often starts with general assumptions about my identity and genitalia, but I often end up giving a science class too.

Some folks noted that more effort goes into the conversations when there's a romantic element to the relationship:

I am married to a straight cis man and came out as nonbinary after we had been married for a number of years. At first it was uncomfortable knowing he saw me as a woman and sexualized certain parts of my body that I didn't want sexualized. But I realized that a lot of the discomfort was because I was labeling those parts of my body myself. There was a learning curve, with lots of conversation about how he sees me and how I see myself. We now have the understanding that we are just two humans together, and we can let go of societal labels and expectations. It has freed up our sex life in a really comforting, beautiful way.

If Partnered Sex Triggers Dysphoria

IF YOUR PARTNER isn't seeing and affirming you during sex, or your dysphoria is getting in the way, there are steps you can take to increase your comfort and pleasure.

I find how my partner perceives me is INCREDIBLY important. If I can feel them putting me in the "woman" category in their brain, I do not feel affirmed. And then my dysphoria gets so much worse.

Having sex with a trans partner who is conscious and aware of my gender dysphoria triggers is incredible. I've explained it to cis people before but I feel like they never "got it." The first time we had sex I told my partner that certain words for my genitals really turn me off and they understood without explanation.

In any context, at any point, you're always allowed (and encouraged!) to stop any sex that doesn't feel good to you, for any reason. Sometimes having a safeword for moments like this can be useful (see page 278 for more about safewords). Establish with your partner a word that means you stop all sexual activity, and set boundaries about what happens next. If you need all touch to stop until you feel comfortable again, or if you need to be held and comforted, a safeword can help make that happen. Putting yourself and your own needs first like this might feel intimidating to some people, and you might experience guilt about interrupting what your partner thought was a good time. But I know that if I were having sex with someone who was uncomfortable, I'd want to know as soon as possible to see whether we could fix what was wrong. Give your partner the benefit of the doubt, and guess that they would want to know too.

BDSM and Kink

BDSM BASICALLY MEANS playing with pain, power, and/or sensation. The letters stand for bondage, discipline/domination, sadism, and masochism. This kind of sex can be seemingly mild, like having your partner blindfold and then arouse you, passionately running your fingernails down your partner's back, or asking a partner to hold your wrists down while you have sex. Or it can involve more intense play and sensations, like using a whip, handcuffs, or candle wax. The most important thing is that both partners agree about what they want to do—like every kind of sex, what's highly arousing to one person may be a total turnoff to another. It's the norm in BDSM communities to have detailed conversations well before any play starts, defining what each partner wants and what each person's boundaries and limits are. BDSM does not need to involve sex, orgasm, or nudity and often does not.

BDSM can be thought of in at least four overlapping categories:

○ **Bondage**, which could mean being tied up with rope, handcuffs, neckties, and so on, or asking a partner to hold you down. For some people, choosing to give up power and control to a trusted partner can be super arousing.

○ **Impact play**, which could include spanking, floggers, whips, spatulas, and similar toys. People who enjoy this kind of play might be turned on by the pain or the intensity of sensation, as well as the experience of being dominant or submissive.

○ **Sensation play**, exploring sensations that can feel good and release endorphins, ranging from feathers, ice cubes, or silk scarves to biting, clothespins, or nipple clamps. Blindfolds might be used to intensify the sensation.

○ **Domination and submission**. Regardless of what you and your partner choose to do, for many people the experience of consensually giving power to their partner, or taking power over a partner, can be both sexy and exciting.

Kink, on the other hand, is typically defined as anything outside the bounds of more "conventional" sexual behaviors, like the ones in the titles of most of this book's chapters. It's an umbrella term that can encompass an infinite universe of activities, including BDSM, role-playing, fetishes, voyeurism, exhibitionism, leather, and many more. While the list of kink "categories" can seem surprising or titillating, interest in kink is more common than you might think: some studies find about half of adults are interested in it. And our friends who own sex toy stores tell us they see sales increasing, especially items related to bondage and power play.

Kink and BDSM are enormous subjects that deserve far more space than we can give them here. If they appeal to you, or they're already part of your life, we encourage you to find the websites, books, social media, and in-person communities where you can learn, explore, and continue to enjoy, safely and consensually!

Giving up control of my body to someone else is a huge turn-on.

Cuckolding. I love it because it makes my partner come off as desirable to other people and makes me more attracted to them as a whole.

I have a pregnancy fetish. I don't want children but I find pregnant women very attractive and the risk of getting pregnant when having sex turns me on.

I enjoy humiliation, but it's something I have to set clear boundaries with. Make sure your kinks don't diffuse into everyday life in a way that will make you uncomfortable.

Hair pulling—it's a nice way to be controlled without too much pain.

My only kinks are, like, being watched or being surprised by my partner finding me masturbating.

Safewords: The Sexual Pause Button

PEOPLE WHO CHOOSE sex play that involves pain or power generally agree on a "safeword" with their partner. (This kind of sex also requires that both people consent and not be drunk or high.) If either partner says the safeword, it means both people promise to stop right away and check in. A safeword is a word no one would ordinarily use in a sexual situation, like "armadillo," "mashed potatoes," or simply "safeword" itself. Once you've agreed on a safeword, you can struggle against the silk scarves you asked your partner to tie you up with, or play out a dominant/

submissive fantasy where one of you bosses the other around sexually, or enjoy the intense sensation of being flogged just the way you wanted to be, knowing that if you say your safeword, the action will stop immediately. Some kink play involves gags where a person might not be able to speak. One option is "tapping out," a term used in martial arts. The person being choked firmly pats their partner two or three times, indicating it's time to release the gag or hold. Others agree on a gesture like making jazz hands or some other easily noticed motion.

The person who says the safeword or uses a safegesture might just need a small adjustment ("Can you retie that scarf on my left wrist? It's pinching a little.") before the scene can continue. Or they might need a change of plan ("This is getting pretty intense for me—let's cuddle for a little so I can catch my breath."). People who enjoy BDSM say that having a safeword and a trustworthy partner helps them feel safe, relaxed, and even lets them thrash around and say, "No, stop!" if that's part of their fantasy, knowing there's a surefire way to actually stop the action if they want to.

9

Coming with Pride
A Few Extra Notes for Lesbian, Bisexual, Queer, Asexual, Intersex, Transgender, and/or Nonbinary People (and Their Partners)

One of the awesome things about the subject of orgasms is that it's about your body, not your sexual orientation. For the most part, an orgasm is an orgasm. Although body parts, types of stimulation, and the meaning of the experience vary from person to person and situation to situation, the biological reflex is essentially the same no matter who you are or who you do.

Since sexual pleasure and orgasms are equal opportunity, our approach throughout this book has been to explore the range of how bodies work and how to increase the odds of experiencing pleasure, regardless of who you are. Take oral sex, for instance: If you have a clitoris, the same basic concepts apply no matter the gender of the person with the tongue—or the gender of the person with the clitoris, for that matter. Anybody (with any body) can enjoy the hum of a vibrator in just the right spot. Both cishet (cisgender heterosexual) and queer people sometimes find it challenging to have an orgasm. Information about how clits like to be touched doesn't vary whether one flies a rainbow flag or not. Many people who've had partners of more than one gender say sex is a similar experience regardless of the gender of the person you're getting it on with—that the person matters more than the genitals or the identity.

That said, there *are* unique topics that arise for queer, trans, and nonbinary people that aren't covered in other chapters. Here's our chance to dive into some of those!

When Sex Involves Two Vulvas

SOME THINGS ARE different when vulvas-owners have sex with each other. The person on top, for instance, can push their knee hard up against the other's crotch for the bottom partner to grind against, a move that would likely elicit howls of pain if the one on the bottom had a penis. Two partners with the same parts can compare their orgasms—and each other's "performance" at the identical activities—more directly than partners whose bits differ. And without a penis in the bedroom, there's no assumption that the night will end with intercourse, tab A in slot B.

For the purpose of finding a common language, we'll sometimes call sex between two people with a vulva "sex between queer women" or "lesbian sex." We know that not everyone who has this kind of sex uses these words—some may identify as heterosexual, asexual, curious/questioning, or use some other word. And, of course, trans women who happen to have a penis may be having "lesbian sex" too.

Part of the value in talking about "lesbian sex" for all of our readers is that we get so many questions about it. While other questions' frequency waxes and wanes over the years, the question "How do lesbians have sex?" remains a mainstay. What folks are really trying to figure out is how it's possible to have sex without a penis. The question reveals the flawed but widespread assumption that sex equals a penis in a vagina—which makes it impossible for many to imagine sex with, say, two vaginas and no penis.

As readers of this book know, the best sex is about *way* more than just a penis in a vagina; it involves hands and fingers, lips and tongues, breasts and nipples, labia and clitorises—not to mention the more than fifty other body parts people named on our survey when we asked for their favorite erogenous zones (page 32). Lesbian, bi, and queer people with a vulva are just as likely to have every one of

A Few Words About Language

MAYBE SAYS: THE term *lesbian* and the expansiveness of queerness can make this topic difficult to discuss. What many people think of as "lesbian sex" could also be seen in a "heterosexual" couple (if a transgender man is with a cisgender woman, their sex might involve two vulvas). Likewise, there are lesbian trans women, but if they have a penis, their sex life might look quite different from what we're discussing here. And there are nonbinary and trans masculine people who feel strongly attached to the identity of lesbian, while rejecting the identity of woman. Also, plenty of cis women who have sex with women don't identify as lesbians—they might call themselves bi, pan, gay, fluid, queer, and so on. All of this is to say that "lesbian sex" can mean an infinite number of things to different people. We know and acknowledge that "lesbian" does not equal two women and does not equal two vulvas. However, when most people ask how lesbians have sex, they're really curious about what happens when a penis isn't in the equation. So, we're going to do our best to be expansive in our language, while acknowledging that it's not a perfect fit for everyone.

those body parts as anyone else, and it's not difficult to combine them in ways that feel fantastic. For people who love penetration (some do, some don't), fingers do a great job. You can vary the thickness by changing the number of fingers, and fingers can curl and place pressure in ways that penises can't. Dildos—worn as strap-ons (see page 235) or used by hand—are an option too.

There isn't anything unenjoyable about being sexual with a woman. I love everything. Rubbing, tasting, stimulating her breasts, kissing her whole body, oral sex, fingering. I love it all. Sex with women is slow, patient, and exciting. The payoff for all the work and energy is the intimacy and moaning.

I love exploring someone's body and taking my time. I love breasts. I love my own breasts as well as other women's. Kissing another woman is one of the most sensual experiences of my life.

I LOVE being with women! It's like a sexual awakening for me. I love kissing all over her body. I love touching her for hours. I love using my hands and mouth, or a toy, whatever. It's about the emotion involved. Even when we're being rough and dirty, it's still about the love underneath it all.

Some queer women also remarked on how hot it can be to touch your partner's body and be able to imagine *exactly* how it feels to be touched there. Some said the "forbiddenness" of queer sex can make it feel extra sexy, or that being with a same-sex partner can make it feel safer to "lose control" during sex.

And the Challenges

THAT SAID, SEX with another queer woman isn't all sunsets, roses, and orgasmic perfection.

I think the biggest challenge is that not all women are the same. Just because you're turned on by rough penetration doesn't mean your partner is. You have to really communicate about it. Also, there's always the fear that she might be better than you at something. Like what if my partner really turns me on when she's using her tongue to stimulate my clitoris, and I do the same to her and she doesn't react?

I'm used to boys, I don't know so much what to do to girls.

Even though I have all the same parts, I didn't know what she liked or disliked, and was afraid of doing something wrong. I wanted to be good, but I ended up being scared.

When I first kissed a girl, I wasn't sure what to do with her boobs. Mine are pretty compact and hers were the real deal and I had no idea how she might want to be touched or even what you DO with them.

Others who took our survey observed:

○ Flirting with, asking out, or otherwise finding a same-sex partner can be tough since there's less of a social script about how to do it—and because you sometimes have to guess if a given woman would be flattered or offended to be asked out by another woman.
○ Some women find it challenging to be sexually assertive, or to find a partner who is. Relationships between women sometimes lack a sexual initiator.
○ Compared with pleasuring a partner with a penis, it can be harder to help a partner with a vulva and clitoris have an orgasm and to know whether your partner came.
○ Some women feel guilty about having sex with other women because we live in a homophobic society that's uncomfortable with and sometimes hostile toward same-sex sex and relationships.

Queer women also have to deal with the reality of homophobia in their lives. One nineteen-year-old woman commented on our survey, "I am constantly worried my family or someone from my hometown will find out and I will be disowned or killed because of it." It's not uncommon for LGBTQ people to fear or experience violence. For more resources and support about this kind of violence, as well as same-sex sexual assault and domestic violence, check out the National Coalition of Anti-Violence Programs at https://avp.org/ncavp/.

Hands and Mouths

WE ASKED OUR lesbian, bi, and queer women survey respondents what were their favorite ways to be pleasured by a same-sex partner. Unsurprisingly, the summary of the hundreds of data points could be boiled down to two words: *oral* and *fingering*.

Oral sex was head and shoulders above the rest (pun intended), with 61 percent of the respondents mentioning it as one of their favorite activities.

I love getting oral. So soft, smooth, it just feels incredible and I get lost in it.

I like that they know what they are doing and how it feels and looks.

Also ranking high were fingers and hands, with 30 percent mentioning them. Some people specified using them for clitoral stimulation, some said they liked them for penetration, some mentioned both, and some didn't say. Fingers and hands are the Swiss Army knife of queer sex: they can do almost *anything*.

Fingers! I enjoy both penetration and external simulation. I like it so that way I can still kiss/hold my partner while it happens.

Other high-ranking activities: using vibrators, dildos, and other toys; kissing and making out; grinding; and touching all over one's body. Check out the chart on page 286 for the full menu of activities that multiple survey respondents named as their favorites.

What I love about whole body touching is that it is special. Since I'm not a nudist, and I'm easily cold, I reserve my whole body naked touching to the special occasion of sex. But more than that, feeling with my body feels different than feeling with my hands. It adds to the experience because it can be all-consuming.

I love kissing and grinding for a long time until I'm super turned on and then having her go down on me while she fucks me with her fingers.

One other difference between queer and cisgender heterosexual sex is that queer partners seem less concerned about making simultaneous orgasms a goal, and more inclined to alternate and take turns. That allows each partner to devote all their energy and focus at a given moment to either giving or receiving sexual pleasure, without trying to do both at once. It's also a generalization and an oversimplification. Queer partners certainly sometimes both receive pleasure at the same time and can aim for simultaneous orgasm if they wish. Cishet partners can and do take turns. And many people of all genders and sexual orientations find it pleasurable to pleasure their partner. But if one considered only the overall averages, taking turns giving and receiving pleasure is an LGBTQ strength.

When your partner also has a vulva, what are your favorite ways to be pleasured?

KEEP IN MIND that these were the *favorite* activities, so even the ones that appear to rank low are some people's favorite way to spend time with a partner! And of course, most people include many of these in any one sexual interlude. One person's reply about their favorite way to be pleasured: "All of them? Is that an okay answer? Lol. Hands, toys, mouth... everything." The good news is sexual pleasure is an all-you-can-eat buffet—you're allowed to choose "all of the above," as long as you have a willing, consenting partner!

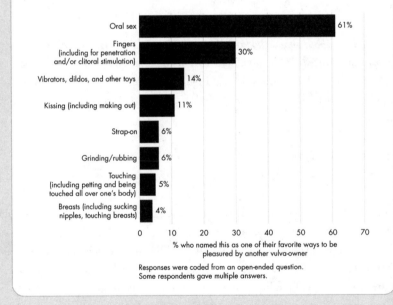

	%
Oral sex	61%
Fingers (including for penetration and/or clitoral stimulation)	30%
Vibrators, dildos, and other toys	14%
Kissing (including making out)	11%
Strap-on	6%
Grinding/rubbing	6%
Touching (including petting and being touched all over one's body)	5%
Breasts (including sucking nipples, touching breasts)	4%

% who named this as one of their favorite ways to be pleasured by another vulva-owner

Responses were coded from an open-ended question. Some respondents gave multiple answers.

Lesbian Sex Secrets

IF YOU'RE GOING to be rock and rolling, you'd be wise to take to heart these tips from those who have gone before you:

1. Cut your nails. While there are exceptions to every rule, vagina-owners generally want their partners to have smooth, trimmed fingernails. Fingers and hands can be at the heart of the action when two vulva-owners sleep together, and being stabbed between the legs by a daggerlike talon isn't pleasant. Some say the fastest way to distinguish between "lesbian" porn featuring women *pretending* to be lesbians and porn featuring the real thing is to check out the length of the fingernails. (If you're a femme who loves those acrylics, a workaround is to put a cotton ball on the tip of your finger and then put on a nitrile glove for finger-to-vulva play.) Some also leave most of their fingernails long, and just trim those on their dominant pointer and middle fingers.

I enjoy using my hands to have sex with a woman. I enjoy most any sexual act with a woman, but using my hands I'm the most comfortable and have had the best results.

2. The journey may be the destination. The process of enjoying each other's bodies, touching and being touched (or licked, sucked, stroked, fingered) is the main point. Breast play or oral sex isn't just "getting ready for the real part," it *is* the real part. (Of course, this can be true for couples of any combination of genders and parts.) That means it can go on as long as you want. If you're both enjoying it, be creative and get lost in the pleasure.

3. Rediscover the joy of grinding. Many people with a vulva find that rubbing their body against their partner's body is pleasure all its own. Rubbing your clits together can hit both of your most sensitive parts at once. Your breasts can rub against each other at the same time. There's even a special word for this type of grinding, *tribadism* (nicknamed "tribbing"), but a lot of people who partake just call it delicious.

I love being humped by a woman (though I HATE that word—it makes me think of dogs humping the legs of strangers). I think I really enjoy it because of the pressure on my pubic bone, and the feeling of moving together with someone in a kind of rhythm.

What About Scissoring?

SCISSORING IS A sex act that involves two vulva-owners interlacing their legs as if they were two pairs of open scissors and grinding their vulvas or clitorises together. But you already knew that. Since becoming a common porn scene, scissoring has experienced skyrocketing interest—especially in straight people's imaginations of how lesbians have sex.

Among Certified Lesbians™, there's far less interest in scissoring, mostly because there are so many other easier, more effective ways to stimulate your partner's vulva and clit. Does scissoring happen? Yes. Do some people enjoy it, essentially as a tribbing position? Absolutely. Three percent of our survey respondents listed it as their favorite activity when with a same-sex partner. But this is one sex act where the cultural imagination of its popularity far exceeds the reality. Feel free to give it a try, whether or not you and your partner both have a vagina—any kind of genital-on-genital rubbing can feel good, and you may revel in how well your bodies fit together. But if you give up, sweaty and possibly having pulled a muscle in your thigh, to return to more tried-and-true fare, well, you won't be the first couple to do so.

There's something really amazing about grinding with a woman. It's just pure, unhampered, skin-to-skin, sensual fun.

4. Call your own shots on penetration. Whether you like the sensation of having something in your vagina—or you don't—is about as personal a preference as whether you sleep on your side or your stomach. Among queer vagina-owners, penetration is totally optional. (It's optional for straight vagina-owners, too, but they often face way more pressure to have penetrative sex. In reality, all partners, of all genders and sexual orientations, need to make sure they're on the same page.) Your partner's never liked penetration? No problem! You can make their clit sing. You love the feeling of something inside you, the bigger, the better? The two of you can have a good ol' time shopping for the biggest purple silicone schlong you can find. Of course, fingers and hands can work great for this too. Your partner may enjoy a finger or two inside, unmoving, to have something to squeeze against, but may not like the feeling of in-and-out thrusting. It's totally up to you; your Queerness Quotient doesn't hinge on your opinion about having anything in your vagina.

We use sex toys quite frequently and have dreams of building our own sex palace/ dungeon! My partner [is trans] and, thus, we do a lot of acts that could be interpreted as heterosexual (blow jobs, penile-vaginal/anal intercourse). Of course, we do these all with the aid of a harness and dildo.

5. Be smart about safer sex. It's a myth that queer women aren't at risk for HIV and STIs. It's true that HIV risk is lower for two vulva-owners having sex with each other than for those sleeping with penis-owners, but it's not zero. Plus, there's no shortage of STIs that those with a vulva can inadvertently share with their partners through skin-to-skin contact (like grinding, described earlier), vaginal fluids, menstrual blood, or sharing sex toys. You're not off the hook in the safer sex department just because pregnancy isn't a risk.

6. Most aspects of sex between queer women are in every other chapter of this book. Lesbian, bi, and queer sex is about the clitoris and all the great things you can do with it (Chapter 1), masturbation (Chapter 3), oral sex (Chapter 4), G-spots and squirting (Chapter 6), sex toys (Chapter 7), partnered sex (Chapter 8), and anal play (Chapter 11). Enjoy!

> ### For More on Lesbian Sex
>
> *GIRL SEX 101* by Allison Moon
> We're endlessly impressed with this book and its inclusivity of trans folks. It's fun to read, comprehensive, and as accepting and nonjudgmental as a good friend dishing up sex advice.

When Orgasms Aren't Happening

RESEARCH FINDS THAT compared to heterosexual women, lesbians average more orgasms, more frequent orgasms, more multiple orgasms, and are more likely to have orgasms the first time they have partnered sex. Great news, right? Absolutely!

But here's the catch (yep, there's always a catch). It's common for queer-identified sex partners to internalize a sexual goal of one orgasm per partner per interlude. Once that goal has been achieved, it's time to get up and figure out what's for dinner. (Maybe you've heard the old joke: "Why do people have orgasms?" "How else would we know when to stop?") Of course, sex doesn't have to lead to an orgasm every time for each partner, and sexual or sensual pleasure doesn't have to end after the orgasms unless you want it to.

We find that lesbian, bi, and queer people with a vulva who haven't had an orgasm, or who find it challenging to do so, can end up feeling like underachievers, as if one's attendance at a Pride march should automatically make orgasms flow freely. Knowing that 86 percent of lesbians say they usually or always orgasm during sex (compared with 65 percent of heterosexual women) makes it that much more demoralizing if you're one of the 14 percent who don't. The reality is that having a partner with a vagina is no guarantee of having an orgasm—and not being able to "give" your partner an orgasm doesn't give you an F on your Queer Report Card. Some people, no matter what their sexual orientation, need to touch their own clit or use a vibrator during partnered sex to be able to get off. That's the reality of how some bodies work, not a sign of some shortcoming on the partner's part.

Likewise, some vulva-owners of all sexual orientations have a body that just hasn't made the orgasm connection yet, for a myriad of reasons or no reason at all, as we explored in more detail in Chapter 3. A small percentage of queer women who are not able to come say doing so isn't important to them. Some say that for them, the thrill of sex is pleasuring their partner. Their sexual high point is their partner's big O.

One dynamic is nearly impossible to avoid when people with a vulva have sex with each other: orgasm comparison, and sometimes orgasm competition. Given the orgasmic diversity in the universe, it's unlikely that both orgasms will be the same in any given relationship or interlude. More likely, one person's climaxes will be faster and the other's slower, one's will feel stronger and the other's weaker, one's will go on and on while the other's slip by in the blink of an eye.

The solution? Well, it's unlikely two people are going to become orgasmic twins, no matter how hard they try. (Of course, cisgender heterosexual couples also frequently have gaping differences between their orgasms, but they typically write these off as "men and women are different" and don't expect otherwise.) Two vulva-owners may feel compelled to experiment to see whether new approaches could help the "lesser" orgasms get stronger, longer, or more likely to go from zero to sixty in 3.9 minutes. But rather than stressing too much, it's probably best to acknowledge and embrace the fact that their sexual responses are different—not better or worse.

Disclosure and Transitions

WE WANT TO take a moment for Maybe to focus on two topics that are more specific to trans and nonbinary people: disclosure and medical transitions. They've been popping in throughout the rest of the book, but we're going to spend the next few pages exploring some topics that most cisgender people don't have to think about.

Disclosure

Disclosure, what some people might call "coming out," is a person's decision to tell others about their identity. For trans and nonbinary people, disclosure before sex and intimacy can be especially tough to navigate. Some people have no choice in the matter: they have to disclose because they're not assumed to be cis. Perhaps their gender presentation isn't in line with cis-centered standards, or maybe they know their body will look different than what their partner might expect when clothes come off. Others won't feel safe being intimate unless their partner understands their identity. For some people, their decisions about disclosure are impacted by intersectional identities: Black trans women experience disproportionate levels of antitrans violence due to the intersection of racism, transphobia, sexism, and socioeconomic status. Given this reality, disclosure must be a deeply personal decision.

> *I don't feel comfortable being with a sexual partner who doesn't know such an important part of me. It has limited my potential partners, but I don't feel safe trusting my body to someone I can't trust with my gender.*

For some, not disclosing means running the risk of having their partner misgender them. A casual partner might assume they are the gender they were assigned at birth and treat them accordingly. Other trans people are often assumed to be cisgender and could navigate intercourse without being misgendered or needing to disclose anything.

I stand very firm in the belief that it is each person's decision when, how, and if they disclose details about their identity. After hearing myriad experiences from other trans and nonbinary people, I find that each person knows what's most comfortable and feels safest for them. I reject the notion that people are liars or deviants when they don't tell their sexual partners that they're trans, and I refute the claim that disclosure is a requirement. Remember: Trans people wouldn't be considered liars for not disclosing their identity if everyone wasn't assumed to be cisgender.

There have been times in my life when I didn't feel safe enough to come out, and that felt scary, being so close to someone who didn't know about it and wondering how they would react if they found out.

There are limitless different ways to disclose, and limitless reasons why some people choose not to. Some people don't want to open themselves up to a line of invasive questioning when they're just aiming for a quick hookup. Others might not consider their gender identity to be the most important thing about them, and might want someone to get to know them before knowing that they're trans.

If you have a choice whether to disclose or not, it can be helpful to think through questions like:

○ Do I expect this to be onetime sex or a more ongoing sexual relationship?
○ Do I know whether this person is cis? Trans? Nonbinary?
○ Do I have any reason to believe this person might not respond well?
○ Am I prepared for a potentially negative or unfavorable response?
○ How comfortable will I be if I don't disclose?
○ How comfortable will I be if I do disclose?

Whether my partner is a trans person or not determines if I come out as trans to them. I have never come out as trans to a cishet partner.

At heart, disclosure is not only rooted in each person's comfort level but also in their perceived safety and trust. Given the risk of violence trans people face from intimate partners, disclosure decisions can literally be a matter of life and death.

Medical Transitions

Some transgender and nonbinary people take hormones like estrogen, testosterone, antiandrogens, and progesterone, to affirm their gender and offset dysphoria. Some don't. Some trans folks have gender-affirming surgeries or procedures: top surgeries, bottom surgeries, or other procedures. Although these surgeries too often become the topic of cis people's obsessive curiosity, trans people know they're only one piece of who they are—possibly important to themselves, possibly irrelevant. Plenty choose never to have surgery, or are unable to access or afford surgery.

Since sexual response, orgasms, and pleasure are so intricately tied to genitals and hormones, it's not surprising that people's experience of orgasms and pleasure often change if hormones, surgery, and/or other elements of medical transition are part of their life. It can take time to relearn how to experience pleasure or have an orgasm (or learn for the first time, if you've never had an orgasm before).

Bottom growth has changed how I need to stimulate myself to reach orgasm. There has been a lot of trial and error to get the right technique.

I have had a meta [metoidioplasty, a type of surgery to create a small phallus] done. There is a significant difference in sexual pleasure and orgasms. I found that I ended up with the greater intensity typical of males while retaining the longer length of orgasms typical of females.

I definitely had to re-learn how to make myself come because my body was changing so fast. I'm currently taking a break from testosterone (for family/financial/safety reasons) and now I'm having to learn all over again how my body works!

Some people notice physical changes, both positive and negative. Many of our trans masculine survey respondents who'd had top surgery (removing breast tissue

Why Are We Talking About Medical Transitions?

MEDICAL TRANSITIONS CAN look a lot of different ways, and the way a person transitions should be completely up to them. You don't need to have surgeries to take hormones, and you don't need to medically transition at all to be trans. We're going to take some time to talk about medical transitions here because they're a big topic that sets trans and nonbinary people apart from cisgender folks, not because we think it's a required part of being transgender. We'll be focusing mostly on hormones, top surgeries, and genital surgeries, since these are most likely to impact sexual pleasure. This focus doesn't mean that other forms of affirming surgeries aren't important, but they don't tend to change much about pleasure and orgasms, aside from making one feel more at home in one's body.

These aren't onetime, one-moment decisions: for many of us it's an evolution as our lives, identities, situations, access, and the world around us evolve too. The individual reasons why each trans and nonbinary person makes the choice to transition the way they do could fill another book (and have!). For some starting points for books, websites, and social media accounts, visit iloveorgasmsbook.com.

to result in a flatter chest) expressed sadness at the nipple sensitivity they'd lost, sometimes as an unexpected side effect. But some had the reverse experience with sexual nipple sensitivity. There are also some folks who have their chest touched for the first time after surgery, now that they're comfortable enough to do so. Others commented on the ways other body parts had changed:

My bigger clit has made things easier, I would say. The target is easier and it's easier to use a range of toys.

My voice change made me more comfortable making noise.

I used to be able to get off just by having my nipples and areolas touched. Now I have a lack of sensitivity in my chest because of top surgery. It may as well be a piece of plywood on my chest; I don't feel a thing and it kind of makes me sad. However, what I lack in nipple/breast sensitivity has been well made up for by my underarm sensitivity. Like it migrated there or something.

Before top surgery, I had to be binding continuously during sex, and I had no erotic nipple sensation. Now, I can be completely bare to the skin and scars, and both my partner and I can touch my chest—I don't have to avoid certain positions or motions because they'd make me aware of my chest. Also, despite still having large areas of reduced touch sensation, I actually have erotic sensation in my areola and nipples now. It's truly amazing how much of a positive change happened.

Since I experienced significant bottom growth due to testosterone, my clitoral orgasms are so much more intense. It feels like I touched a lightning rod when a clitoral orgasm hits.

For some, orgasms themselves feel different after or while medically transitioning—and for others, not at all. It makes sense that feeling more grounded and at home in your own body would lead to more pleasure. But it's not always a matter of finding more or less pleasure; sometimes people find whole new ways of experiencing pleasure.

It's hard to aptly describe, but orgasms are more full-bodied waves instead of like pinpoint release now. I'm much more sensitive now and my orgasms build more slowly and then wash over my body. I'm also much louder now.

Since starting T [testosterone], they feel a lot less intense and are localized in my genitals instead of being a full body experience.

HRT [hormone replacement therapy] has changed how my body experiences different stimulation. Wand vibes are my best friend now, and I like nipple stimulation a lot. And other areas of my body are much more sensitive in general, like my thighs, neck, and tummy.

I'm a lot hornier, I have wet dreams now, I jerk off a lot more, and my orgasms are longer and more enjoyable.

I've always been told orgasms are different on HRT, but personally I've never really noticed a difference.

Some people noticed a change in the emotional side of sex, or what sex means to them. Being more in touch with one's body can cause a shift in the ways we connect emotionally, especially during something as physical as sex. But also, hormones influence our emotions, so it's understandable that some people's connection to sex and intimacy changes with their hormones.

I used to feel much more emotionally invested in sex, and now it seems more functional to me, so I feel less affected by what happens during the act. I've also learned to listen to my body differently, which has in turn made me a more adventurous partner.

Having sex now, post-top surgery, is like a whole new world. It's insane how much more confident and in my body I am—I'm so much more present and eager to receive affection.

I hated my body with every bit of my soul. I couldn't bathe myself and could barely change underwear. That didn't keep me away from sexual arousal, but the guilt I felt after doing it made me feel sick to my stomach. It's only after years of hormonal treatment and beginning to feel more comfortable with myself that I stopped feeling guilty.

Many trans or nonbinary people who sought and feel good about their medical transition choices find they're simply more comfortable having sex—and therefore are more likely to experience pleasure—as their body more closely reflects their authentic self.

Sex after top surgery was just so much better. I was like, OH wow, that was really holding me back!

Being nonbinary has freed me from the expectations I'd put on myself to act a certain way. I used to be very self-conscious of looking or sounding a certain way while I orgasmed, thinking that partners would expect me to be this high-pitched, squeaky coming person. I love a good hard moan and groan, and love being loud as hell.

I just like sex more now that people don't see me as a woman. I read as male but identify as genderqueer. My body tells a gender story that is not binary, and I love that. I choose partners who value me and my body and that makes me hot. Testosterone was a key part, but not the only thing.

Asexuality and Orgasms

YOU MIGHT THINK asexuality doesn't belong in a book about sexual pleasure. You'd be wrong! *Asexual* (some use the shorthand "ace") is a word for someone who doesn't experience sexual attraction. Although ace people are not drawn to other people sexually, they may still experience arousal, and some (though certainly not all) are orgasm enthusiasts. When thinking about orgasm and asexuality, the key is to separate out sexual attraction to *other people* from enjoying or experiencing pleasure *in one's own body*.

Asexuality is a broad umbrella. Some of the more common ace identities include:

○ **Aromantic:** someone who experiences little or no romantic attraction to others, possibly satisfied with friendships and other nonromantic relationships
○ **Demisexual:** someone who doesn't experience sexual attraction unless they form a strong emotional connection with someone
○ **Gray-asexual, graysexual, Grace, gray-A:** someone who exists in the gray area between allosexual (a person who experiences sexual attraction) and asexual

About half of ace people masturbate regularly. They may have what's called "nondirected desire," meaning that they feel sexual desire but have no interest in sharing arousal or orgasms with another person. That self-pleasuring may result in orgasm, or it may be pleasure for the sake of pleasure, without orgasm as an end goal.

I enjoy giving myself orgasms and have little desire to engage with a partner sexually. I get the job done on my own!

I get pleasure from masturbation but I don't know if I've orgasmed or not. I've been masturbating since I was a little kid, as far back as I can remember. I'm still asexual because I don't desire sex with others, and sexual imagery is not what makes me want to masturbate.

Some asexual people choose to be in relationships and pleasure their partners sexually, even though they don't have sexual attraction for them. Still others more closely fit what many might guess: a general disinterest in orgasms and sexual pleasure.

Orgasms aren't a big part of my life. Sex isn't a big part of my life in general.

I honestly don't care if I ever have an orgasm. I've been told that I should care, and that orgasms are great and it's sad I've never had one, but I don't feel like anything is missing from my experience of sexual pleasure. I don't have a goal of orgasming when I decide to seek sexual pleasure.

In recent decades, a rich asexuality community has formed around the world. Asexuality.org (the Asexual Visibility and Education Network) is a great starting place to find your way to all things ace: podcasts, books, social media accounts, research, and more.

Intersex Experiences

INTERSEX PEOPLE HAVE internal or external anatomy, hormones, and/or sex chromosomes that don't fit the binary categories of male and female. Intersex bodies are part of natural human diversity and are generally perfectly healthy because genitals, hormones, internal anatomy, and chromosomes can fit together in many different ways. Even if an intersex person's body is different from what people typically expect, most of the time there's no need for medical intervention. Yet shame and stigma about these differences result in the medical system changing people's bodies through invasive surgeries when they're too young to understand or consent, usually before age two. Parents may feel pressure to "do what the doctor says," and may not even be aware that there are other approaches. Intersex is about *biological* differences, and that makes it different than transgender or nonbinary, which is about *gender identity*. You can be trans *and* intersex because gender identity and sex are separate categories.

For example, most people are born with either XX or XY chromosomes, and a vagina or penis, respectively. But that's not the case for everyone. Some people are born with only an X chromosome (called XO), or get an extra sex chromosome, like XXY. Other people are born with "ambiguous genitalia" that isn't clearly a penis or a vulva; they might have characteristics of both. The outdated and inaccurate term for that condition was "hermaphrodite," which is now considered a slur. These days, the word *intersex* is used to describe this wide range of conditions that can indicate these types of bodily differences. An estimated 1.7 percent of people are born intersex, roughly the same percentage of people worldwide who have red hair.

I was born without external genitalia—I didn't have a clitoris, vagina, or penis. Due to my confusion about my sexuality and gender identity, and my self-consciousness about my body, when I was growing up I declared that I wouldn't date or marry. But in the last year, I've realized that sex is something I can enjoy, after all, despite my background. I'll need more surgery at some point to have "normal" vaginal intercourse, but my boyfriend and I make it work. When he stimulates the area where the entrance to my vagina will be with his fingers or penis, I usually climax fairly quickly. Being in this relationship has been good for me—it's given me hope that I can be sexually satisfied, and I can provide satisfaction for someone else, even with my physical differences.

One of the biggest factors affecting some intersex people's orgasms is whether they had medical interventions like genital surgery as an infant or toddler. Some doctors perform medically unnecessary surgeries to make a child's genitals look more "normal," with no regard for what effect this might have on the person's future sexual pleasure. For example, a doctor could remove part of a baby's clitoris if it's believed to be "too long—too much like a penis." Although the clitoris may look more "average" after the surgery, that baby just lost some of the most sensitive nerve endings in the body. How could that *not* have an impact on sexual pleasure and orgasms later in life?

I've had two, maybe three, experiences that resemble the descriptions of spontaneous orgasm. This has been the only pleasure available to me so far. I was born with a full female reproductive system and genitals, but also an ambiguous organ that might have been either a large clitoris or a micro-penis, and half a male system. The doctors never checked for female organs, and at the age of three they closed my labia and covered my possible clitoris in a skin graft. They imagined I should be a boy. Puberty arrived in my mid-twenties, primarily female with some extra androgens. I have a vagina with lots of sensation, which would be almost normal except that its opening is the width of a straw. I have almost no clitoral sensation. I do have desires, and I wish there were a way to indulge them. But no doctor anywhere is willing to touch my case because I'm not a child anymore. There is a hell—it's located at a hospital in Baltimore. Don't do this to your kids.

One additional burden and challenge for intersex people is that many don't realize they're intersex. Some are aware that something about them is different, but don't know the word *intersex* and aren't aware of the existence of an identity and a vibrant community. Since surgeries commonly happen when children are so young, parental discomfort or shame sometimes results in intersex youth and adults being unaware of or unclear about what happened to them.

The intersex movement's message is clear: Unless there's a medical emergency, keep doctors' scalpels away from children's genitals. Many intersex babies are still assigned male or female at birth, and they figure out the rest as they go. Parents also have the option to raise a child as free from gendered expectations and constraints as they can, and let the child find their own path and identity. Then, once the person is an adult and more aware of who they are, they can choose to have surgery to change the appearance of their genitals, or not.

Intersex people born with ambiguous genitalia who were lucky enough to have escaped childhood genital surgery are often the ones who say their sex lives are the most satisfying, because nobody interfered with their genitals or damaged their nerve endings. In most cases, their genitals work just fine for purposes of pleasure.

There are entire books and websites devoted to intersex issues; if you're interested in reading more, check out interactadvocates.org (InterACT), which maintains an extensive website with links to intersex groups around the US and the world.

If Your Partner Is Trans or Intersex

IN OUR MANY conversations with transgender and intersex people and their partners over the years, a few themes emerge consistently about being a respectful sex partner of a trans or intersex person:

- Ask, ask, ask...There's no way to know what your partner likes and is comfortable with without talking about it.

- ...But don't turn every sexual encounter into Transgender or Intersex 101. There's a difference between asking your partner what feels good for them and asking them to give you a vocabulary lesson. There's a time and place for partner education, but sometimes it's time simply to play or snuggle.

- Use the trans or intersex person's affirming pronoun, language, and words for their genitals. Follow their lead.

- Realize that some people may not want certain parts of their body touched sexually, or may want them to be touched only in certain ways. Asking how a new partner likes to be touched is always good manners—and even more important when your partner is trans or non-binary. For instance, a partner might perceive a trans masculine person to have breasts, and begin to caress them the way they have caressed cisgender women's breasts. But the trans person may not want their body part touched this way, or at all.

- Likewise, for a trans feminine partner, the part they call their clitoris might look like a phallus to a new partner. They might prefer to have that body part stimulated with one or a few fingers, like any other clitoris, rather than "hand job style" with a whole hand.

- Be willing to let go of some of what you already know about how to please a partner, and be open to finding creative ideas together.

- Once you figure out what sexual activities you and your partner enjoy, have fun! Don't worry about what identity labels you need or how these might change. You'll figure that out over time.

10

Penisology

When it comes to orgasms, penises are rather effective at providing them to their owners. It's virtually unheard of, though not impossible, for a person with a penis never to have had one whereas it's quite common for people with a vulva to find themselves in this situation.

Likewise, during partnered sex, penis-owners do fairly well in terms of orgasms. One study compared orgasm rates among heterosexual, gay, and bi men and women, all cisgender, asking respondents whether they always or usually had orgasms during partnered sex. Ninety-five percent of the heterosexual men said yes, followed by 89 percent of the gay men, 88 percent of the bisexual men, 86 percent of the lesbian women, 66 percent of the bi women, and 65 percent of the heterosexual women. Statistics like these are why this book centers the experiences of people with a vulva.

But there are plenty of penis-owners out there who find things aren't working as they would expect, leading to confusion, disappointment, and fewer orgasms. We asked our survey respondents with a penis whether they've ever had challenges; you'll find a breakdown of their responses on page 304.

This chapter is devoted to solutions for each of those situations as well as other common issues penis-owners face. This chapter's narrow focus on penises sets it

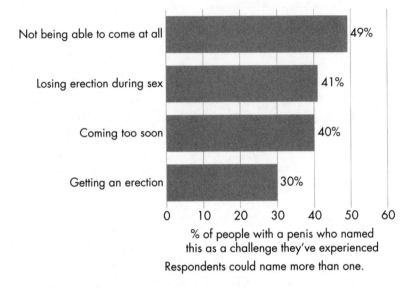

Penis Challenges

% of people with a penis who named
this as a challenge they've experienced

Respondents could name more than one.

apart from most of the rest of the book. However, based on our research, the issues we explore here are the ones on the minds of most people with a penis when it comes to their pleasure and orgasms.

The biggest obstacle penis-owners and their partners are up against has nothing to do with penises themselves: it's an issue of expectations. Our culture leads people to believe penises are perfect machines, always at the ready to get hard and stay hard. While the drug Viagra and its competitors brought heightened awareness of "erectile dysfunction," they've reinforced the belief that if you can't get hard anytime anywhere, there's something wrong with you that needs to be fixed. And though the drug is designed to counteract the natural effects of aging, it's also sometimes used by a younger demographic of penis-owners looking to party all weekend, and by porn stars needing a competitive edge. Viagra has only added more weight to the performance expectations on penises.

Despite how common—in fact, nearly universal—"imperfectly behaved" penises are, few, if any, of the topics explored in this chapter are mentioned in high school sex ed classes. And whether due to shame, embarrassment, or cultural taboos (probably all three), penis-owners rarely discuss them with one another.

Each of the following challenges is unique, but they all have one thing in common: The penis isn't working the way its person wants or expects it to. Many penis-owners grow up with the idea that they should always be able to perform, even if they're feeling ambivalent or just not in the mood.

Most people with a penis have early experiences of orgasm and ejaculation via masturbation. Now, masturbation is one of America's favorite pastimes, and it's perfectly healthy. But sometimes all that "hands-on training"—often using the same technique that reliably produces a fast orgasm each time—doesn't translate perfectly to sex with another human being. One can get a sense of this by comparing it to penetration.

KEY DIFFERENCES:
SEX WITH YOUR HAND VERSUS PENETRATION WITH A PARTNER

	YOUR HAND	PENETRATION WITH A PARTNER
Naked Partner	Usually no other naked person involved, unless you count the images you're streaming on your screen.	Your partner is hot, naked, and wants you! The sheer thrill of it can lead to premature ejaculation. Or stage fright can make it difficult to get hard or come.
Time	As fast as possible, please, before your roommate comes home. Many penis-owners find they can come in two to five minutes or less if they want to.	If you get hard as soon as you get turned on, and have a long sex session with tons of foreplay, you may want to stay hard but not come for a long time. Or you may not be able to come at all, even when you want to.
Arousal roller coaster	Ready, aim, fire! A smooth climb to the top.	Your mission looks something like this: Build up enough sexual excitement fast to get hard and stay hard throughout foreplay; definitely be hard enough to put on a condom.

	YOUR HAND	PENETRATION WITH A PARTNER
Arousal roller coaster *(continued)*		Then, you start having penetration, possibly the most exciting part of all, and your li'l cyclops is enveloped by all the pleasurable sensations of being inside your partner—but, uh oh, now you have to change gears so you don't come too fast. When you're having sex, arousal can involve a lot of loop-de-loops.
On the mind	A desire to come and maybe a fantasy to help.	"Hot damn! We're doing this!" That *it'smyluckyday* feeling can lead to lightning-fast ejaculation. But at the same time, you may be thinking, "What if my partner gets pregnant?" "What if I catch something?" "Am I hurting my partner?" "Is my partner enjoying this?" or any of a trillion variations of "Where is this relationship going?" or "Was having sex with this person the right decision?" All those kinds of (perfectly reasonable) conflicting thoughts can work against staying hard and coming when you want to.
Technique	You've had plenty of time to perfect your skills, and you can stick with the same basic technique—as fast as you want—from beginning to end.	Rushing straight through penetration, with constant jackhammer thrusting, risks being a recipe for a frustrated partner and/or a faster finish than you intended.

I ♥ ORGASMS

With all this in mind, of course penises don't always do exactly what you want them to, particularly when partnered sex is on the agenda. It's totally normal for perfectly healthy, young people with a penis to sometimes come sooner than they want to or not be able to get it up or get off; more than 78 percent of the penis-owners who filled out our survey said they'd run into at least one of these challenges at some point. If this stuff happens occasionally, don't worry about it.

I don't view these as challenges! They are just a natural part of sex.

If there's a partner in your bed at the time, there are plenty of other ways to pleasure that person, including using fingers or a phallic object for penetration if that's what your partner was looking forward to. If one or more of these challenges is becoming a regular occurrence, and that's bothering you, check out the tips below.

So Many Ways to Come

THE TOPICS EXPLORED in this chapter are ones that frequently arise during sex that involves penetration, typically vaginal or anal sex. But please don't forget that there are *many* ways to pleasure a penis. Oral sex is a popular choice, of course. But another underappreciated genre of penis pleasure is rubbing: in between breasts, butt cheeks, or thighs, or between nearly any body parts that work for you and your partner! Penises can rub between the lips of a vulva without penetrating inside the vagina. Curvy partners' bodies often have rolls and crevices that are perfectly suited for penis pleasure. And don't forget the humble hand job. All of these ways of getting off can be great for situations when time is tight, when a partner is tired or not in the mood for penetration, to eliminate pregnancy risk when a partner is fertile, or just as a way to spice things up and get out of a sexual rut.

Advanced Penisology: A Troubleshooting Guide

Challenge: You Can't Get It Up

THE CAUSES OF "erectile dysfunction" can be either physical or psychological. For most people with occasional problems in this arena, the sexual episode in question involved one or more of these factors that make it more difficult to get an erection:

- ○ You were drunk.
- ○ You had an intimidatingly hot partner.
- ○ You'd already ejaculated once or more earlier that day.
- ○ It was a hookup, and you were nervous or uncomfortable since you didn't know the person very well.
- ○ There weren't any condoms available.
- ○ You were exhausted, stressed out, or just plain nervous.
- ○ You were in a rush.
- ○ You were on a medication that affects arousal or erections (common for many antidepressants, as well as other medications).

Or it could have been nothing at all—sometimes an erection will play hard to get (or should that be soft to get?) for no reason.

The last thing to do when you can't get hard is to panic because that creates even more performance anxiety the next time you have the opportunity to knock boots. If you can see that some of the factors on the list above may have been the culprit, that'll help you change your strategy (or at least better understand your body's responses) next time. You can also try relaxing and enjoying the sensations that feel good without worrying about whether or not you get hard. Sometimes the erection shows up when you're just enjoying yourself and not trying to make it happen.

> *Don't obsess about it. Relax. Don't force it and don't get nervous about it. Usually if I just lie down, put my arms around my girl and gently kiss and touch her, I can get my dick back in the ring.*

Typically, this happens when I've been drinking: "whiskey dick." I've found the best way to solve it is just not to drink as much.

Foreplay is the best solution to this for me. I used to go in once my erection was good enough to go in, or had just reached its peak, and I'd rush things. Most guys don't want foreplay because they have no self-control and can't wait to start intercourse. However, I find the longer I wait, the better it is for both of us.

If you have difficulties getting hard, erectile dysfunction drugs can seem like an easy solution. But those drugs bring with them health risks, including sudden hearing loss and vision problems, and potentially a higher risk of skin cancer. We'd far rather see people—particularly young adults—find and confront the roots of their sexual challenges rather than become dependent on pharmaceuticals.

If getting an erection is a consistent problem for you—during partnered sex and alone—then it's worth asking a doctor to rule out possible physical causes. These can be wide-ranging, including hormonal imbalances, thyroid problems, medications you're taking, sexually transmitted infections, or chronic illnesses like diabetes. Also, check out page 314.

Even for older adults, Viagra and Cialis may be emphasizing the wrong thing, says Melanie Davis, author of *Our Whole Lives: Sexuality Education for Older Adults.* "They can create mechanical hard-ons, but can't create desire or fix crappy relationships. People who [take Viagra because they] want their 17-year-old-selves back are facing serious cardiac risks. We need to normalize that erections come and go with age."

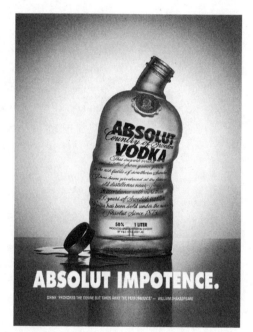

Even Shakespeare knew that, as the *Macbeth* quote at the bottom of this image reads, "[Drink] provokes the desire but takes away the performance."

Challenge: You Come Sooner Than You Want To

For all the talk about erectile dysfunction drugs, coming too soon is an even more common problem. A few tips on how to troubleshoot this one:

○ If you come faster with a new partner because you find them really hot, say so! Your partner will probably be flattered to hear how much they turn you on. This kind of problem may resolve itself as the newness of the relationship wears off.

○ If your partner has a vulva, remember the power of the tongue. Yes, it can be a point of pride to last a long time. But there's a difference between your ego and your partner's orgasm. For most vulva-owners, clitoral stimulation is what it's all about, and that has little, if anything, to do with how long you last. If your partner has an orgasm before penetration begins, as often works so well, then you don't have to worry about "lasting" at all; you can come at whatever point is most pleasurable for you.

> *Cunnilingus gives me a chance to relax and focus the sex act on my partner for a while. Once she's satisfied, it doesn't matter if I finish in ten seconds or forty-five minutes. The pressure to "perform" just goes away.*

○ Come earlier in the day. Many penis-owners have figured out that if they masturbate before a date, that'll slow them down that night.

○ Wear a condom. Sometimes that small decrease in sensation is exactly what you need.

○ Try an encore. Some people with a penis, especially younger ones, find that if they come too fast the first time, they're ready to go again fifteen minutes later—with a lot more stamina in Round Two.

○ Take a break from whatever activity (intercourse, oral sex, etc.) is so physically pleasurable for you, and do something else for a while (maybe pleasure your partner) before returning to it.

> *It helps me to try a less animalistic position. The thrill of doggy style makes for quick coming, whereas many sitting positions are pleasurable but less hormonally thrilling.*

○ Relax and actually tune in to the sensations in your penis rather than tensing up or trying to avoid thinking about how it feels.

This sounds cliché, but being really relaxed allows me to perform longer. I've found that when I'm really anxious about things (personal life, work, etc.) I can't concentrate on the sensations, and I'll come before I realize I'm coming. It seems like the times I'm most stressed out are when I end up being a ten-minute wonder.

○ Learn ejaculatory control by knowing your "point of no return." Because penetration can be an incredibly stimulating experience physically, visually, and emotionally, penis-owners sometimes rush headlong toward orgasm. They race up the mountain—only to tumble head over heels down the other side.

Learning to Last Longer

Some try to stave off their orgasm by concentrating on something completely nonerotic, like doing math problems in their head or thinking about sports. As a college student, Marshall used to bite his tongue, theorizing that pain was the best distraction of all. Many penis-owners find that while that works for a while, they're ultimately fighting a lost cause. Rather than sidestep the problem with these techniques, it's better to address it head-on.

The key is to learn to identify the point when you've neared the top of the orgasmic mountain, the moment when you're on the brink of having an orgasm, without actually having one. Here's how to train yourself:

First, practice when you're masturbating. Most penis-owners speed through masturbation, eager to have an orgasm. Instead, take your time. Sex researchers and therapists William Hartman and Marilyn Fithian found that if you perfect the skills to be able to masturbate for fifteen to twenty minutes before having an orgasm, you'll be able to last as long as you want during intercourse.

During this period of twenty minutes, there may be times when you feel like you're really close to having an orgasm. Don't stop stimulating yourself entirely, but back off just slightly, easing up on the intensity of your touch. When the moment passes, continue the stimulation again. Repeat this process, always paying close attention to the experience of being close to coming, but figure out how to move through that with a lesser degree of stimulation until the "I'm gonna come" feeling subsides.

Once you've mastered this technique during masturbation, you can apply what you've learned to penetration. If you feel yourself approaching the point of no return, slow down or stop moving inside your partner. Consciously slow your breathing. Relax all the muscles in your body, particularly those in your legs and butt. Doing so can work wonders for your ability to last longer. Strengthening your PC muscles with Kegel exercises (they're not only for people with a vulva!), described on pages 34–36, 38, and then squeezing when you want to slow yourself down, can also help.

> *I just take it slow now and don't try to "go for broke" quickly. As my girlfriend puts it, "It's a marathon, not a sprint." She also is more accepting of the fact that sometimes I just need to stop thrusting to regain control.*

> *The easiest way to slow yourself down when you're on top is to give her a long passionate kiss and stop moving altogether for a second.*

Challenge: Can't Get Off (it takes too long to come, or you can't come at all)

This was the most common challenge identified in our survey, with 49 percent of penis-owners saying they'd wrestled with it at least occasionally. As we've said to the vulva-owners who are dealing with an equivalent issue, this needn't be a crisis; anyone can have a great time without always having an orgasm.

> *If I can't or don't feel like coming, it's okay, because sex is about the entirety of the experience to me. Now, sometimes this doesn't work for my partners so I have to reassure them that this isn't an all-the-time thing, and that there will be other days—trust me!*

> *We've spent time talking about our rhythms and I've been more vocal about asking for what I need. We've also discussed that it's okay for one of us not to come every time we have sex, which has helped ease some of the pressure.*

Numbing Creams or Antidepressants?

IF YOU STRUGGLE with coming faster than you'd like, the world of numbing creams and sprays may appeal to you. We don't recommend them. They reduce your ability to enjoy the physical pleasure of sex; they might reduce your odds of being treated to a blow job; and most important, they don't solve the underlying problem—which is totally solvable.

Along the same lines, since antidepressants (specifically SSRIs) are known for making it more difficult to orgasm, sometimes doctors prescribe them to nondepressed patients only for the purpose of slowing down a penis-owner's ejaculation. These haven't actually been found to be that effective (typically adding only a few minutes), they add a host of potential side effects, and, like a numbing spray, they leave you reliant on buying something to have the kind of sex you want.

Use the techniques described on page 311—practiced on your own or explained in more detail during a few sessions with a sex therapist—and most likely you'll be able to master the ejaculatory skills you need to avoid spending your hard-earned cash on prescription meds or trying to numb yourself.

One thing to consider is whether you're putting too much focus on just one part of your body. Like vulva-owners, a lot of people with a penis find that a broader approach to arousal can help build the whole-body momentum to push them over the edge to orgasm. We were struck by the survey respondent who said that "having a massage before, as part of [sex]" helped with the challenge of not being able to come at all.

Many penis-owners in this situation have already tried everything they can think of to make themselves come: receiving oral sex, fantasy, positions they find particularly sexy, dirty talk, and more. Sometimes those are just the ticket—and sometimes not. As with any sexual challenge that's bothering you, if this is a regular experience you're not able to resolve on your own, you might see a doctor to rule out any physical causes. Some prescription medications can be the source of the problem, as can drugs like alcohol, ecstasy, or amphetamines. Multiple penis-owners who filled out our survey said the thing they'd discovered that helped them most was cutting back on the amount of alcohol before sex, as best summed up by one: "Don't drink so much. Mature."

When it comes to psychological causes of not being able to come, one major factor is what author Michael Castleman calls the "delivery boy attitude." If you have a delivery boy mentality, you take great pride in your ability to please your partner; you want to be thought of as an excellent partner who has the skills to "deliver" the orgasms.

If this sounds like you, you have every right to be proud. You've probably right-fully received praise on your lovemaking skills, and as fans of providing pleasure, we shake your hand! The problem is, the delivery boy attitude can trip you up when it comes to your *own* orgasm. By conditioning yourself to be a long-lasting sex machine, ready and willing to provide the pleasure your partner wants, you may be neglecting your own pleasure. Let go of the myth that the ideal penis-owner is focused only on giving partners an ideal sexual experience. It's okay to be human, to enjoy sex simply for the sake of your own pleasure. It's okay to be vulnerable in front of your partner and let yourself go.

If I'm doing something other than focusing on being pleasured, like fondling her breasts or stimulating her clitoris, it's very hard for me to come.

I put all kinds of pressure on myself. I have to remind myself it's not all about her—I'm supposed to have a good time, too. If I'm not enjoying myself eventually it's going to screw up the vibe.

If you're having trouble coming, it's also possible that your penis isn't getting the stimulation it's gotten used to from your self-loving technique. If you grip your penis with your own hand harder than any vagina ever could, try experimenting with using a lighter, slower touch. If you first discovered how to masturbate in an unusual or unique position, you might want to increase your versatility by exper-imenting with other positions that are more similar to the experience of having

Trans Folks and Penises

MAYBE SAYS: THE topic of penises for trans and nonbinary people encompasses many different experiences, types of anatomy, and comfort levels. For starters, trans and nonbinary people often use language for our genitals that might not be consistent with how they'd be labeled in a medical textbook. So, when a trans or nonbinary person uses the word *penis*, *dick*, or *cock*, what they're referring to might look like what a textbook would call a clitoris. Likewise, you might see genitals that look like what that textbook would call a penis, but the owner refers to it as their clit. Using language like this helps many trans and nonbinary folks to reclaim their body and define themselves.

For trans masculine people who take testosterone, "bottom growth" is when that body part gets larger and might start to resemble a scaled-down version of a textbook penis. Regardless of its size and whether or not the person is on hormones, some trans masculine people like to have this body part touched and stroked, in the same way a person who was assigned male at birth might like it. Some trans masculine people might use a dildo and/or harness as their dick.

Some trans masculine folks have bottom surgery to construct a phallus. Others have what is essentially an enlargement of the part that's already there. There is a wide range of surgeries that a person might choose, and an even wider range of what sexuality and pleasure might look like afterward.

Trans feminine people may have the penis they were born with. Some enjoy using it for sexual pleasure; for others involving it in sex can activate intense dysphoria, which can restrict or interrupt pleasure. Using a phallus for sexual pleasure doesn't always have to be insertive in penetrative sex. Some trans women and trans feminine people find a lot of pleasure from rubbing and stimulating their girldick the same way you would a clit.

Also, depending on hormones and other circumstances, trans feminine penises might operate differently than this chapter describes. Playing with different ways to explore pleasure and climaxes could be full of endless possibilities.

Some trans feminine people choose to have bottom surgery to create a neovagina, in which case they'll no longer have a penis. Most neovaginas look and function similarly to the other vaginas talked about in this book, but again, there is a range of experience with pleasure after surgeries.

your penis inside your partner's vagina or anus, even if they're less pleasurable initially. It's fully possible to "train" yourself to respond to and enjoy a variety of kinds of physical stimulation using techniques similar to those described for vulva-owners on page 101.

Challenge: Losing Your Erection During Sex

We saved this one to discuss last since so many of the preceding troubleshooting tips, including not being drunk, help with this challenge. This one's closest cousin is not being able to come at all, since the same dynamics that make it difficult to get off also make it difficult to get the pleasure you need to stay hard. A lot of survey respondents told us that this was one where the connection (or lack thereof) to a partner can make a difference.

> I find my body checks out when I don't feel seen or valued by my partner. To me, these are indicators of the union not being a match in that moment. Or I decide that we need to pause and talk to each other or massage each other or look into each other's eyes. If we can connect from a different angle, then the physical can kick back in.

Honestly, cuddling with my partner and stroking each other's bodies while intertwined and telling each other all of the things that turn us on about the other builds back up that arousal.

Several survey respondents also said that changing positions helped them.

A Few Inches (of Text) on Penis Size

SETH STEPHENS-DAVIDOWITZ IS a data scientist whose career's focus is what can be learned by combing through search engine data. What people type in the Google search box, is, after all, a pretty good reflection of what's on their mind, particularly for problems where Google might just know the solution.

His findings on searches about penis size are dramatic:

○ Nine of the ten top searches by men that include the phrase "my penis" are about size-related concerns, with the top three being "how to make my penis bigger," "how to make my penis longer," and, puzzlingly, "how big is my penis?"

○ Men are 170 times more likely to search for information about their own penis than women are to search about their partner's penis.

○ According to Stephens-Davidowitz, "Men Google more questions about their sexual organ than any other body part: more than about their lungs, liver, feet, ears, nose, throat and brain combined."

Need More Detailed Troubleshooting Help?

WE'RE BIG FANS of the author Michael Castleman, who wrote *Great Sex: A Man's Guide to the Secret Principles of Total-Body Sex* as well as *Sex for Life: Everything You Need to Know to Maximize Erotic Pleasure at Any Age.* Castleman's research is excellent and his advice to cisgender straight men is the best we've seen.

A sex therapist can also be a game-changer. Find one near you at aasect.org.

If you're concerned that your issues might have a medical cause, schedule an exam, and ask your doctor if it might be appropriate to check your testosterone level, thyroid function, luteinizing hormone, and PSA level. In some cases, especially in older people, erectile issues can be a symptom of more serious disease like clogged arteries, so an exam can be a life-saving move.

A Few Words for Partners: Secrets of the Penis

A WELL-KNOWN CARTOON portrays vulva-owners' sexuality as a complex machine, full of dials, switches, gauges, lights, and whistles. The other half of the cartoon supposedly represents penis-owners: a simple on-off switch.

Despite penises' reputation for simple predictability, the system that orchestrates erection, orgasm, and ejaculation is definitely *not* a simple switch but is as wonderful, mysterious, and sometimes complicated as its clitoral equivalent.

If you encounter a partner whose penis isn't working exactly the way either of you had hoped or expected, don't worry about it. Just as you wouldn't want your partner to have a crisis if your orgasm is nowhere to be found on a given day, it isn't helpful to have a crisis over a noncooperative penis. In fact, if your partner suspects that you're upset about it (based on your desperate measures, questions, accusations, or tears), that'll increase their own anxiety, creating the risk that the problem will grow because now you're both stressed out about it. Especially if it's something that happens only occasionally, your best bet is to let them know that as far as you're concerned, it's not a big deal. Don't make the mistake of believing your partner's erection is a good barometer of how they feel about you.

Why all the anxiety and interest in this subject? Porn is a well-hung source. Walking around in the real world, it's obvious some people are taller, others shorter; some have bigger breasts, others smaller. But the penis is a part of the body that isn't normally on display—except in porn. And porn star penises are a statistical anomaly. Studies find the median erect penis is 5.1 inches, with 50 percent of all penises measuring in the 4.7- to 5.6-inch range. Only 5 percent of erect penises are longer than 6.2 inches, and 1 percent are longer than 9 inches, common lengths of porn penises.

In the real world, does it matter what size you are? First, let's be clear: small penises can provide just as much pleasure to the penis-*owner* as large ones. But what do their partners think? In the course of our work, we've informally polled thousands of people with a vagina, by anonymous survey during online events, by show of hands at gatherings in giant theaters, and in breakout groups in lecture halls. First we make clear that not everybody has had sex with a penis or wants to. But for those who've experienced penetration with more than one size of penis and have an opinion, we offer three possible answers:

1. Bigger is better. I genuinely find a big penis more pleasurable.
2. Small is beautiful. I find big penises uncomfortable or painful.
3. Penis size really isn't a significant factor in my pleasure. It's not the size of the boat, it's the motion of the ocean.

The responses we get are close to identical regardless of where we go:

○ About 10 percent always choose category one and say a big penis really feels more pleasurable to them.
○ About 5 to 10 percent say they prefer a smaller penis because a larger one can be uncomfortable.
○ Everywhere we go, 80 to 85 percent say penis size really, truly, honestly has no impact on their pleasure. When we ask, "So are you saying that what your partner does with their hands, fingers, lips, tongue, and words affect your pleasure more than the size of what's between their legs?" the room fills with snaps and applause.

Penis-owners, what does this mean for you? If you have a big penis, hopefully you can find a partner who will be thrilled to discover you. But if you're walking into sexual situations thinking everything you need to please any partner is between your legs, you may be setting up yourself—and your partner—for disappointment. Demonstrate to your partners that you realize your "third leg" is only one of the many ways you're ready and willing to provide pleasure.

If your joystick is on the smaller side, know that there are plenty of partners in the world who would be downright relieved to find you—nearly as many as

What About Gay Men?

THERE'S SOME EVIDENCE to suggest that on average, cis gay men tend to be a bit more size-ist when it comes to their penis opinions than cis straight women. But if you're average or smaller, don't despair. While the gay hookup scene may tilt a bit more toward the superficial, when people are in the market for longer-term partners, most are interested in the whole package of who you are, not just the package in your underwear.

are hoping to find an above-average peen. Be reassured, too, that nearly all people with a vagina who have sex with penis-owners would choose a skilled partner with any size penis over a clueless one with a cockasaurus. There's plenty throughout this book to help you become the kind of partner people brag to their friends about.

And if you're kind of average, well, so are most people! Don't waste your time and money on pills, pumps, lotions, weights, or exercises to make you bigger; none of them have been proven to make any permanent difference, and many risk damaging your body. Remind yourself that penis-owners tend to care more about penis size than their partners do, and choose to spend your time focusing on the things that are far more likely to matter to your partner.

A Partner's Guide to Uncircumcised (Intact) Penises

THE CHANCE THAT a person dating penis-owners will encounter one or more intact ones has changed dramatically over the last fifty years. Since the high of about 85 percent in 1975, the rate of newborn circumcision has fallen to approximately 60 percent today, with wide regional variations. By comparison, in most of western Europe, fewer than 20 percent of babies with a penis are circumcised. So as a partner, your parents or grandparents may never have seen or touched an uncut penis, whereas nowadays, if you're a sexually active adult who meets a bunch of penises in your life, there's an excellent chance one or more will be intact.

First, a word about words. *Circumcised* means a penis that's had part of it (its foreskin) surgically removed. So, rather than describing some penises as "uncircumcised," defining them as *not* having had something removed, we use the word *intact* to refer to a penis that still has all its original parts.

So, what to do with one if you're feeling inexperienced? Well, it's always fine to ask! "Uncut" would be the sexier language to use, as in, "I actually haven't gotten to be with an uncut guy before—maybe you could give me a little demo?" It's a great opportunity for a mini-body tour (see page 261). But you needn't be intimidated—it's still a penis! You might also want to jump right in and try some things, and check in with your partner as you go! Here are some tips.

- Be gentle. Intact penises have more nerve endings than circumcised ones. In general, it will feel better to use the foreskin to slip up and down over the head of the penis rather than stimulating the head directly.

- Foreskins can be fun to play with, and as long as you're not too rough, many foreskin-owners enjoy having them gently tugged, stretched, licked, and so on. During oral sex, you can experiment with putting your tongue under the foreskin.

- Most intact penis-owners like to slide their foreskin back (or have their partner do so) before putting on a condom.

- Especially if you're considering oral sex without a condom, it can't hurt for the penis-owner to wash first, since it's an easy spot for sweat and dead skin cells to build up (kind of like under larger-size breasts). Showering together as part of foreplay is always an option.

- As with all partnered sex, try some different things, listen to your partner's sounds, breathing, and words, and use "which feels better?" with two options to learn what they like.

- Intact penises may not need as much lube, especially for hand jobs or rubbing against body parts. The foreskin's ability to slide up and down acts as a kind of built-in lubrication. That said, the "wetter is better" approach that's savvy for most kinds of partnered sex remains true for intact penises too.

- Since intact penises are in the minority in the US, some of their owners can feel insecure. If you enjoy your time with one, honest compliments are probably especially welcomed. (But that's true for *all* honest compliments about *all* body parts.)

- Have fun! Uncut penises are just as healthy and hygienic as circumcised ones, and have more potential ways to play with them. Enjoy the explorations with a consenting partner!

11

Knocking at the Back Door
Advice for the Anally Curious

Anal sex: Just the inclusion of this chapter in a book on orgasms has some people thinking, "Awesome!" while others are shaking their head, "Oh, really?"

In many ways, a chapter on anal sex is a perfect match for a book like this. It's a sex act that many people are curious about, lots try at least once, and that can feel considerably better with preparation and education. How you approach anal sex can make a huge difference as to whether it's pleasurable or painful. If it's something you're considering, definitely read these pages so you don't have to learn the hard way.

Anal sex was once stereotyped as "something gay men do." In reality, some gay men do, and some don't. In a study of nearly twenty-five thousand gay and bi men that asked about their most recent sexual experience with a man, only 37 percent reported anal sex.

These days, it's an increasingly common activity among people of all genders and sexual orientations. In a national survey conducted by Indiana University, researchers found that 24 percent of adults had received anal sex (meaning they had been penetrated) at some point in their lives. Rates of receiving anal sex tend to climb as people move from their early twenties into their thirties, gaining sexual experiences along the way. For cis women, the percentage who had been a receiving partner grew from 28 percent as young adults to 46 percent among thirty-somethings. For cis men, it rose from 10 to 15 percent at the same ages. A full 58 percent of fortysomething men had had anal sex as the insertive partner, more than double the 20 percent of 18- to 24-year-olds who had had the same experience. There's less data on trans folks, particularly from large-scale studies, but our survey found that 43 percent had received anal sex at some point.

All the percentages are higher than they've been in the past, perhaps a sign of the increased popularity of butt sex, an increased willingness to admit to it in a research interview, or both.

Anal Sex Around the World

THE UNITED STATES ranks seventh in terms of the percentage of adults who say they've had anal sex, according to the Durex Global Sex Survey. (These percentages are probably somewhat higher than the actual numbers since people who volunteer to fill out Durex's survey may not be representative.) Last on the list? Taiwan, where only 1 percent of people list it among their experiences. Here's the top ten list:

1. Chile 55%
2. Greece 55%
3. Italy 50%
4. Croatia 49%
5. Finland 49%
6. Norway 48%
7. United States 47%
8. France 46%
9. Bulgaria 45%
10. Sweden 45%

Many Ways to Play: Tongues and Toys

ANAL SEX IS the headline grabber, having taken its place alongside vaginal and oral sex as an option for penetrative sex. But there's a lot more to pleasuring an anus than simply penetration.

The anus is dense with nerve endings and lots of people find it can be an erogenous zone. Anal stimulation can be provided by one's own or a partner's fingers (touching around the opening or putting a finger inside), with a tongue, or with sex toys. Some people who like the sensations of having their anus touched also enjoy anal penetration in some form, but find most penises too big to be comfortable.

I find anal sex to be pleasurable, but with fingers or a small dildo. This is because when it comes to anal sex you have to work up to something larger. There are a lot of nerves just dying to be touched.

I prefer anal sex with fingers and we do that all the time, but anal sex with a penis hurts so much.

Rimming, also known as analingus or simply "eating ass"—sexual contact between one person's mouth and another person's anus—has made its way into memes, television, and popular culture. And why not? Most recipients of rimming say it feels pretty darn good. Many people who've tried rimming find it pleasurable, thanks to the combination of the tongue's abilities (which oral sex aficionados know and love) and because the anus is sensitive. Others say to each their own, but they're going to steer clear of putting their own tongue down there. Rimming does carry a risk of transmitting bacteria and STIs like hepatitis A. Plastic wrap or dental dams are effective barrier methods. Considerate recipients of rimming always wash or shower beforehand.

I enjoy rimming my partner because I think a beautiful booty is sexy as hell. So burying my face in a magnificent ass and chowing down is a huge turn-on. I think the somewhat taboo nature of it also adds to the excitement. And, of course, when my partner shows that she's really enjoying it, it's a real thrill.

Tom Brady's End Run

TOM BRADY, WIDELY considered to be the greatest football quarterback of all time, made a splash when he came out as a rimming fan with a single-worded Instagram comment. Another account posted a photo of a hippo appearing to eat another hippo's butt, with the caption, "As soon as bae gets out of the shower #AssEatinSZN." In response, Tom Brady commented, "Yep" with three laughing-crying emojis. His admission rocked the internet, generating thousands of replies. The general sentiment was perhaps best summed up by the comment: "This is how you become the GOAT [Greatest of All Time]. Take notes, boys."

Toys designed for anal play have also grown in popularity. Butt plugs, designed for penetration, usually look like dildos with a base. They often have a narrow top and bottom to allow them to be worn inside, unmoving, rather than sliding in and out. You can use a regular dildo for anal play, too, as long as it has a base. Some people enjoy anal toys that vibrate. Others like anal beads, a collection of beads on a string, because they enjoy the sensation of feeling each bead enter their body. The whole string can be pulled out to intensify the moment of orgasm, or be removed slowly afterward.

I just find that having a dildo or anal plug inside me always amps up the orgasm intensity.

The first time I ever came was the first time I used a butt plug, and that was awesome.

My first time orgasming with anal beads inside me, I was by myself and experimenting. It was a very big orgasm; cum went everywhere. Then I had to clean it up and change the sheets. My wife was very pleased that I cleaned the bedroom and changed the sheets without being asked!

When inserting toys into your anus, keep in mind:

○ **They should have a flared (wider) base, or a handle.** Unlike a vagina, which is a closed-off space that ends at the cervix, the rectum leads into five feet of large intestine. If you accidentally "lose" a sex toy inside the vagina, you can always fish it out again with your own finger, provided you relax enough and experiment with different positions. With the rectum, it isn't so easy to "rescue" lost toys yourself. Anyone who's worked in emergency rooms has stories about mortified patients who needed some nonflared object (most commonly a vibrator without a flared base) removed from their rectum. You can avoid finding yourself in this situation by inserting only objects with ends that prevent them from slipping completely inside.

○ **Use lube.** The rectum doesn't lubricate itself, so lube is essential with anal toys—and anal sex, for that matter!

○ **Check for smooth edges.** Because the rectum's tissue is more delicate than the vagina's, don't insert any objects with rough edges.

○ **Don't go from anus to vagina.** Don't use a toy for vaginal contact after it's been in someone's anus unless you've washed it or put on a fresh condom. Bacteria from the anus can make for an unhappy vagina.

Why Do People Like Anal Sex?

PEOPLE ENJOY ANAL sex for lots of different reasons:

○ Pleasure and orgasms! In our survey, 39 percent of people with a vulva had orgasms during anal sex, and of those 22 percent could get off from anal penetration alone, 24 percent with a combination of vaginal and anal penetration, and 73 percent with anal combined with clitoral stimulation. For people with a penis receiving anal sex, those numbers were even higher, with 29 percent having orgasms from penetration alone, and another 95 percent reporting that a combination of anal and penile stimulation did the trick.

I enjoy anal sex because I know my partner is turned on by it, and having him turned on makes me very turned on. It's always a little uncomfortable, sometimes quite painful, but I still enjoy it, just not too often.

I like anal sex because it's different. It feels good, and I love knowing that it's so tight and pleasurable for my partner. I don't do it very often, which also makes it fun. With my first boyfriend, it was a special something we did when I had my period.

Everyone Has an Anus

ANAL PLAY, WITH or without penetration, can be a great option for trans and nonbinary people who don't have the option of frontal penetration or don't enjoy having their front genitals stimulated. Basically, anal can be a fun gender-neutral choice because everyone has a butthole, and anyone can receive pleasure from having it touched or stimulated.

When I thought I was cishet, I didn't do anything anal, but I also find a sweet pleasure in being submissive. The orgasm when I engage in anal play is phenomenal.

Whether it's an orgasmic experience or not, many enjoy the way it feels. In our survey, 19 percent of the vulva-owners described the experience of receiving anal sex as "very pleasurable," and another 45 percent said it was "somewhat pleasurable." Again, the penis-owners were even bigger fans, with 49 percent considering receiving anal sex to be "very pleasurable" and 44 percent saying "somewhat pleasurable."

I enjoy bottoming! I like my partner to penetrate me, either vaginally or anally. I also love to masturbate solo while wearing a butt plug.

Some penis-owners also reported that they enjoyed the sensation of being on the penetrating end; a partner's anus feels different than a vagina or a mouth around their penis (many who've tried it say not necessarily better, but different).

○ Some people are turned on by the excitement of breaking a taboo, the idea that anal sex is "naughtier" than other kinds of sex, similar to the way many people say they're turned on by having sex in a place where they could be caught.

All the nerves there make it feel good, and because it seems like such a naughty thing, it turns me on more.

○ Some like that there's almost no risk of pregnancy. (See page 335.)

Agreeing to Sex You Don't Enjoy?

IT'S FINE IF you agree to do something you feel "meh" about because your partner really enjoys it. This is a common part of healthy relationships, whether it's watching a movie you weren't that excited to see, waiting patiently in a store while your partner shops a sale, or attending a sporting event your sweetie loves. You might choose this same approach in bed from time to time, having some kind of sex simply because your partner loves it. It's not okay if you're doing something because your partner is pressuring, coercing, or shaming you to do it—that's not consent. The difference is whether you agree of your own free will, and it's important.

Agreeing to do something you're not that into makes more sense in the context of a caring, mutually giving long-term relationship than in a one-night stand hookup. But even in a caring, long-term relationship, you still have the right to say no to what you (or your body) don't feel comfortable doing, and the right to stop at any time.

○ Others don't particularly enjoy the physical sensation of anal sex, but their partner derives so much joy from the act that they like doing it occasionally as a "special treat" for their partner.

I think I mostly enjoyed how much it got my partner off, but also it feels dirty and taboo and that's hot.

Some people feel a special emotional connection during anal sex because the act seems particularly intimate to them.

Prostate Stimulation: A Penis-Owner's Perk

PEOPLE WHO WERE assigned male at birth have a gland called the prostate. It's part of the reproductive system: Sperm travel through it on their way from the vas deferens into the urethra during ejaculation. As they pass through the prostate, the gland helps their cause by contributing prostatic fluid. That fluid is what gives semen its milky or white appearance, and also helps prolong sperm's life if it finds itself inside a vagina. (Statistically speaking, in any given day worldwide most of it doesn't—but that's still the prostate's evolutionary purpose.)

Another fun prostate fact is that its muscles are the switch between urination and ejaculation. Many penis-owners have had the experience of having a really full bladder but being unable to urinate if they're also really aroused. During partnered sex, you might excuse yourself to go use the bathroom, but then find yourself standing in front of the toilet, rock hard and unable to pee. If you've ever been in that situation, or if you've been the partner patiently waiting, you can thank (or curse) the prostate.

Apart from its roles as sperm-supporter and pee-to-ejaculation switcher, the prostate has an additional superpower: it can feel great when stimulated sexually. The most direct way to do so is through anal penetration. You'll find the prostate inside the anus, about two inches inside the rectum, toward the front of the body. If your partner is facing you and inserts their finger inside your anus, they can try the curved "come hither" motion, or try stroking it or just applying gentle pressure. It's a similar process and similar location as finding the G-spot inside the vagina, which is why the prostate is sometimes called the "P-spot."

In our survey, rates of experience with prostate stimulation varied by gender identity and sexual orientation. Only 25 percent of straight cisgender men had tried it, and that number climbed to 82 percent for bisexual cis men and 91 percent for gay cis men. Among trans and nonbinary folks with a prostate, at least 75 percent had tried it as well.

For those who tried it, the reviews were overwhelmingly positive, as seen in this word cloud of some of the common responses:

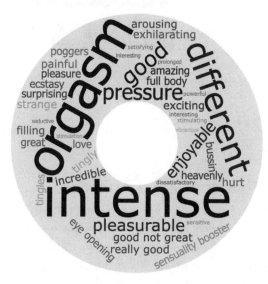

But it wasn't all bliss, as others gave it mixed reviews:

For me, it's a sexual spice, not a main dish. It's not been the sole cause of orgasm, but it can be a nice addition (li'l bit of salt and pepper), or a major distraction when I'm overthinking.

Enjoyable and painful, depending on the experience.

I'm not sure where my prostate is, and I am pretty sure that the pleasure I get from penetrative play is not related. Prostate-specific toys I have tried have almost universally felt physically uncomfortable and not pleasant.

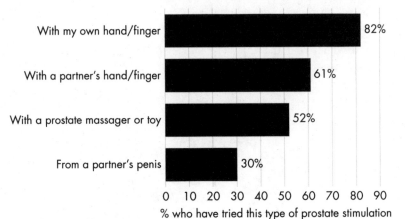

Prostate Stimulators: What's Your Method?

Of those who had experienced prostate stimulation, here were the most common ways they've had it:

Method	% who have tried this type of prostate stimulation
With my own hand/finger	82%
With a partner's hand/finger	61%
With a prostate massager or toy	52%
From a partner's penis	30%

% who have tried this type of prostate stimulation

Essential Tips for Good Anal Sex

[Content note: The first item in this section mentions sexual assault.]

No matter who's on the receiving end, anal sex can be a positive experience, whether or not it's an orgasmic one. But it can also be downright painful and unpleasant if it's not done carefully and respectfully.

1. Make sure both partners are willing and interested. We'll say it again: Everyone has the right to decide what they will and won't do sexually. It's perfectly okay to "just say no" to any sexual activity that doesn't appeal to you, including this one. The partner who's been told no doesn't have the right to badger or coerce the one who's not interested. It's equally wrong for a partner to pretend their penis "accidentally went in the wrong hole" or to "slip it in" sometime when their partner is drunk, high, sleeping, or otherwise unaware—that's rape. Talk about it first, make sure you're both in agreement, and if so, proceed to step #2.

He put it in the wrong hole. I didn't like it and hadn't asked to try it.

Pegging, Prostate Massagers, and Penis-Owners

MANY STRAIGHT CISGENDER men aren't so sure about putting something in their anus, and may even wonder whether enjoying having something up their butt means they're actually gay. The answer is absolutely not! Sexual orientation is about who you're attracted to, not whether it feels good to have something in your butt. And sadly, fears rooted in homophobia prevent a lot of guys from experiencing potential pleasure that's literally part of their own body. But two newer turns of phrase have been a huge boost for straight cis comfort: "prostate massager" and "pegging."

Pegging is the term for when a person's anus is penetrated by a partner wearing a strap-on dildo. The word is traditionally used when the strap-on wearer is a cis woman penetrating a cis man, but there's no reason to limit its use to these genders! It is an invented word, the winning entry in a contest hosted by sex advice columnist Dan Savage for the purpose of finding a word to describe the sex act that previously had no name. It's earned legions of fans, and introduced an entire generation of men to the pleasures of butt sex while avoiding the squirm-inducing words *anal sex*.

I love using a dildo in a strap-on harness on my partner, as it makes me feel a little dominant. Normally I would consider myself a bottom/receiver but I also love to give pleasure, so the dildo is nice for me to fill both those roles during sex.

It's transgressive. And the reversal of power dynamics can be really fun!

There was some taboo-ness to it at first that made it hot, but at this point it's just a unique sensation. Having to dedicate and plan for it ahead of time adds some nice anticipation to it.

Likewise, the phrase *prostate massager* has bolstered interest in toys designed for anal pleasure marketed to cisgender men. They're toys designed to help you reach and stimulate your own or your partner's prostate. Some vibrate, some don't. We think the term sounds so wholesome. Who doesn't want a massage?

I personally don't get pleasure from anal but I do enjoy seeing my partner turned on and enjoying it. He understands I don't enjoy it as much as him, so he lets me initiate it when I feel comfortable doing it.

2. Get relaxed and in the mood. Like vaginal penetration, anal sex works best when you've spent some time making out first, to get in the mood. Most people unconsciously condition themselves to keep the muscles around their anus tight, perhaps providing inspiration for such expressions as someone being a "tight ass" or "anal retentive." You can use the Kegel exercises described on pages 34–36, 38 to get acquainted with the muscles in that part of your body, and learn how to squeeze and relax them fully. (Kegel exercises squeeze and relax both the vaginal and anal muscles; they're all connected.) Figuring out how to relax one's anal muscles can make penetration much easier, and it works better if anal play is something the receiving partner actually desires. If the person is not interested, the anus knows and may not relax, making for painful or uncomfortable anal sex.

3. Start small. If you're ready to experiment with what it feels like to have something inside your anus, start with fingers before you try a penis or sex toy. You can use either your finger or your partner's. The person inserting the finger should follow the same advice we give on page 287 about trimming nails. Put plenty of lube on the finger you're going to insert to make insertion more comfortable and safer.

It took me a long time before I worked my way up to fully enjoying anal sex. It's really hard to relax those muscles enough that you don't feel discomfort. The best thing is to slowly work your way up. For instance, on the first experience try one finger for a little while. Next time try a little longer. Maybe add another finger once that's comfortable, and so on.

4. Use lots of lube and a condom. The most-repeated advice from our survey takers who had received anal sex was a single word: "LUBE." Unlike the vagina, which often gets wet as arousal ramps up, the anus doesn't produce its own lubricant. Therefore, using lubricant for anal penetration isn't optional—it's essential. Lube helps make anal sex comfortable and reduces friction that could result in small tears in the tissue of the rectum. There's more info about lube on page 166. There's no such thing as too much lube when it comes to back door action. A condom is important (unless you're both fully tested and trust each other to have unprotected sex only with each other) because unprotected anal sex is higher risk for HIV and STI transmission than unprotected vaginal or oral sex. Hint: the smoother the condom the better; this is not the time to pull out your prized collection of ribbed and textured condoms.

Because the rectum can contain bacteria that aren't healthy for a vagina, anything that's been inside the anus should be washed (or get a fresh glove or condom) before going into a vagina.

Can you get pregnant by having anal sex without a condom? It's nearly impossible, because sperm would have to make their way out of the anus to the opening of the vagina, and then swim up the vagina. Sperm are ambitious little swimmers, but it's highly unlikely they'd make it that far. Do be careful about getting ejaculate near the entrance to the vagina, though—the closer sperm get, the greater the pregnancy risk.

5. Experiment with bearing down. With the finger, sex toy, or penis right outside your anus, you can try to mimic what you would do with your sphincter muscles if you were pushing out a bowel movement. This motion, known as bearing down, helps your sphincter muscles open up for a moment, making insertion much easier. It helps if what's being inserted is not head-on, pushing directly against the sphincter, but is instead at an angle alongside the perineum. This allows it to slide in as the sphincter opens.

6. Go slow, slow, slow. If you've seen hard, pounding anal sex with no warm-up in porn, and expect to replicate the performance and have both partners enjoy it, you've been greatly misled. Whether receiving fingers, a sex toy, or a penis,

Meet Your Gooch

FOR SOME REASON the quite small, mostly ignored triangle of skin between the scrotum (or vagina) and anus has many names: perineum, gooch, taint, chad, grundle. The medical term, *perineum*, is used for all bodies; many of the others are used more often to describe the body part for people with a penis. The word *taint* is said to have a particularly charming origin: "'Taint the balls but taint the asshole," from a Tom Robbins novel, also described as "'Taint pussy, 'taint arse."

Although the gooch is unlikely to be a magic pleasure button (if yours is, enjoy!), it can certainly be a sensual area to explore on your own or with a partner. For people with a prostate, it can also be a less direct way to stimulate it without penetration.

the anus needs a slow, gentle approach. Start with lots of foreplay, whether it's a massage, touching the outside with a finger, or rimming. Some people find it more comfortable if the sphincter is approached at a slight angle. Once penetration begins, the person being penetrated always chooses the speed and depth of penetration, as well as calling the shots when it's time for a partner to stop moving or pull out. The penetrating partner should be closely tuned in to whether the angle is comfortable for their partner. Because the walls of the rectum can be sensitive, it can take creativity and patience to figure out which position feels best. Pulling out should be just as slow and careful a process as inserting.

Go slow, don't be afraid to warm up, and breathe. I have wonderful orgasms from anal, and in fact had anal before vaginal sex.

Start slowly and communicate with your partner. Tell your partner when it's okay to go in a little farther, when to stop for a moment to let you get accustomed to it. Once you're all the way in, wait a minute and just hold me and comfort me and make sure I'm ready before you start moving again. Talk to me and kiss me on the cheek or shoulder (in a sweet way, not a sexy way). Once I'm ready, start slowly and ask me before going faster or harder.

Bootie Cleaning

POOP IS, INDEED, an inhabitant of the Back Door Continent. Chances are you won't see any if you clean up first, because our body does a great job holding poop fairly high up, not close to the bottom passage where you might go exploring with a finger, toy, or penis. But if crossing paths with a little here or there would be very upsetting, then this might not be the time to visit where the sun don't shine.

You have a few options for how to clean. Mild soap and warm water around the outside of the anus and just a little inside will do the trick, and for many people that's their preference. A baby wipe can serve the same purpose in a pinch. It's an easy approach, especially if ass-eating is your plan, and is also the preference for some people whose play will involve penetration.

Some people choose to anal douche, basically squirting a small amount of warm water or saline into the rectum to flush out any poop. You can do this with a store-bought douche bulb, a Fleet enema (the kind with just saline, not a laxative), a hose attached to your shower (make sure the water flow is gentle and warm, not hot), a baby mucus sucker, or a small ear syringe. Regardless of which you choose, make sure it's clean and well lubricated before you insert it, and time your clean-out routine for an hour or two before your anal play to allow plenty of time for everything you squirted in to come out. You don't need to use much water or spray it very far up; a small amount will do the job.

An anal douche might boost your anal comfort and confidence feeling cleaner before you play. But it also risks causing mild irritation, which is never good before penetration. So, you have to figure out the balance that feels right for you, and that may take some experimentation. If you do choose the douche route, limit it to once a week max. And choosing not to douche at all is common too.

Even if you've cleaned yourself, mouth-to-anus contact brings the risk of STIs, HIV, and hepatitis A, B, and C, so if you and your partner don't know your status,

The Scoop on Anal Numbing Lubes

STAY AWAY FROM products like Anal-Ease (also spelled Anal-Eze), Easy Anal, Ass Relax, and similar numbing agents or lubes that contain benzocaine. Benzocaine is a local anesthetic typically used for topical pain relief. With anal sex, pain is your body's way of telling you that something's not right, that you could be getting hurt or harmed. It's one thing to use a local anesthetic after you've been stung by a bee: You know what happened, the bee is now gone, and you're left coping with the pain. But with anal sex, if something hurts, you should stop and figure out what's wrong, not numb yourself up and push forward, potentially damaging your body in the process. Anal sex done right doesn't hurt. Plus, being numb reduces the possibility that you might actually enjoy it!

it's a good idea to protect yourself by using a dental dam (maybe a flavored one!) or plastic wrap.

As with any sexual activity, some people have powerful orgasms as a result of anal sex, some strongly dislike the sensations, some aren't interested at all, and everywhere in between. Adding clitoral or G-spot stimulation at the same time increases the odds that a vagina-owner will have an orgasm during anal sex, and stimulating other parts often helps penis-owners too. So can figuring out a position that works well for each partner's body.

I've had orgasms from anal sex alone sometimes, but they're much stronger and more likely when my clitoris is being stimulated too.

I'm very particular about anal sex. I only find anal sex pleasurable if there's clitoral stimulation involved and if my partner doesn't expect anything more than slight penetration. There's no "in and out" and no full penetration, just slight entry by the head of the penis.

I love anal sex, but only in a face-to-face position, not doggy style. I lie on my back and hook my legs around my partner's waist, so we're basically in missionary position, except we're having anal instead of vaginal sex. For me, the sensations are really pleasurable and even more intense than vaginal sex. I can have orgasms in this position because his pubic bone hits my clit, plus I think I get some G-spot action internally. I'm a lot more relaxed in this position than from the rear, and I think the angle is better.

Postscript

When the doctor told Dorian she had cancer, she didn't know whether she'd live to see her thirtieth birthday. The possibility of her dying young was terrifying beyond words.

The truth is, none of us know whether we're going to live to be thirty, or fifty, or one hundred. But we do know our lives will be better if we surround ourselves with people we love and respect, who love and respect us in return—and if we care for and respect our body, because it's what we've got as long as we're here. It's incredible, really, the things that bodies can do, and orgasms have got to be among the sweetest.

Orgasms reduce stress, relieve menstrual cramps and headaches, burn calories, reduce junk food cravings, help you sleep better, and are perfect to share with someone you love. Wherever your life's journey takes you, we wish you good health, long life, and plenty of orgasms!

Breast Cancer Action

We're pleased to donate 10 percent of our book royalties to Breast Cancer Action, one of the smartest, savviest organizations confronting the cancer epidemic and working toward true cancer prevention. So far, we've raised over $50,000 through our book and T-shirt sales. To learn more about Breast Cancer Action and get involved, see bcaction.org.

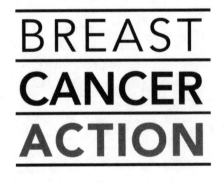

Acknowledgments

We are incredibly lucky to be surrounded by a wise and thoughtful group of friends, relatives, fellow sex educators, and colleagues who gave generously of their time to make this a better book. The number of hours they collectively devoted to the words and statistics in these pages is nothing short of staggering. This book is a thousand times richer and more accurate thanks to their willingness to read draft chapters, fill in stray details, track down research studies, and share insights and experiences from their personal and professional lives.

At the top of this list is Maybe Burke, who has been a dream collaborator, shaping and improving our content on this subject since the moment we first met them. Every sentence in this book reflects Maybe's influence and insights. Their patience, humor, and savvy were indispensable as we wrestled together with the complexities of gender, bodies, and language in night owl Zoom sessions.

We couldn't have asked for a better team of editors: Renée Sedliar's support for this book spans back to its first edition, and her insights on how to update it while keeping its original spirit intact were perfectly on target, right down to the new title. Alison Dalafave's smarts and fresh set of eyes were exactly what the manuscript needed late in the process. Her finishing touches in every chapter were just right. Iris Bass and Cisca Schreefel wisely navigated the book through the final stages of the publication process.

We are deeply indebted to Rachel Dart, Melanie Davis, Schmian Evans, Lindsay Fram, Amy Johnson, Sarah Mell, Michael Oates Palmer, and India Wood, who spent countless hours reading, editing, suggesting, and revising every chapter, and have influenced our work in so many other ways.

Josh Albertson, Ashton Applewhite, Stephanie Campos, Janie Fronek, Alison Hart, Maggie Keenan-Bolger, Skye E. Kowaleski, Mike Mirarchi, Liz Richards, Katy Tierney, Connor Timmons, Kelsey Van Nice, Mary Ward, and Kate Weinberg also contributed significantly and repeatedly throughout our writing process.

We turned to colleagues with specialized expertise on topics we wanted to be sure we got just right. We appreciate the insightful assistance we got from K. Michelle Doyle, Debby Herbenick, Nathan Leonhardt, Karaya Morris, Andrew Pari, Bill Taverner, Lisa Wade, Searah Deysach of Early to Bed, Neena Joiner of Feelmore 510, and Gina Rourke of Nomia.

A huge cheer for LaWanda Johnson, Suzanne Murray, and the 282 Pure Romance consultants who filled out our survey, and for Brandon Maccherone for his work on the book's website. Simon Metcalf and Claire Kinnel saved the day by helping us number crunch our survey results. Our work wouldn't be possible without all the behind-the-scenes support of John Kilguss, Keri Kramer, and Cori Lewis.

Thank you to research and publicity assistants Anji Agarwal, Kehana Bonagura, Jaeda Buchanan, Ari Tamar Gewirtzman, and Nicole Lomax. Shoutouts, too, to Eric Breuninger, Jonathan Kang, Arlene Istar Lev, Julia Nickles, Leon Potik, Haley Robertson, and Aly Mifa Solot for lending a hand with exactly what the book needed at key moments, and to Jocelyn Benson, Laura Briggs, Betty Dodson, Matthew Lore, Melissa Platten, KaeLyn Rich, and Toby Simon for being such an essential part of the journey that led to this book.

Many thanks to our families—we've been asked many times over the years what our parents and other relatives think of our work, and we're thrilled to be able to report honestly that they are big fans.

Last but certainly not least, we thank the tens of thousands of people who have read this book's first edition, attended our educational programs, and participated in our focus groups, and the 3,525 people who filled out the surveys for the book's first and second editions. Your generosity in sharing extraordinarily private experiences, joys, fears, questions, and insights ground our work in the real world. You have taught us more than we ever could have imagined.

Index

strap-on, 143–145, 234–236, 333
submission, 277
surgery: bottom, 155,
175, 223, 293, 315–316;
childhood genital, 299–301;
gender-affirming, 66, 262,
293; on intersex individuals,
299–301; top, 293–297
swing, sex, 149

tabletop position, 148–149
tantric sex, 173
taste, oral sex and, 116–117,
120–121, 132, 140
teledildonics, 108
testosterone, 293, 295, 297, 315
toothbrush, electric, 225, 230
top surgery, 293–297
trans feminine people: clitoris
stimulation, 302; erogenous
zones, 33; masturbation,
105–106; penises and,
315–316
trans masculine people: breast
touching, 302; ejaculation/
squirting, 203; masturbation,
105; penetration, 174; sex
toys for, 223; top surgery,
293–295; vaginismus, 170
trans men, 143, 247
trans women, "penetration"
without penetration, 155
transgender people, 280–302;
anal sex, 324, 328;
antidepressant use, 77;
body tours, 261; coverage
of issues in this book,
8; definition of term, 9;
degendering penetration,
174–175; disclosure, 291–293;
dysphoria as barrier to
pleasure, 74, 84; erogenous
zones, 33; fantasizing
by, 41; gender-affirming
surgery, 66; language used
to describe genitals, 262–263;
masturbation, 105–106;
Maybe Burke's story, 9–11;

medical attention, concerns
over seeking, 170; medical
transitions, 293–297; oral
sex, 112, 124–125; orgasm
advice from, 79–81;
partnered sex, 274–275;
partners of, 301–302;
penises and, 315–316; porn
representations of, 247;
prostate stimulation, 331;
representation in survey data,
15; sex toys for, 223, 231–232;
squirting, 205–206
tribadism (tribbing), 287–288

urethral opening, 63, 64
urethral sponge, 194
urinary continence, 201
urination, urge for, 205
urine, squirt/ejaculate
compared to, 189, 204–205

vagina: arousal boosting, 67;
euphemisms for, 24–25;
examining yours, 63–64;
G-spot (see G-spot); medical
care, 123; neovagina, 316;
penetration, 142–187; pH of,
117, 120; touching yourself
experimentally, 65; use of
term, 23; wetness, 31–32, 45,
70, 166–167
vagina-owners. See also
vulva-owners: ejaculation,
188–190; tips for partners of,
251–259
vaginal orgasm, myth of,
165–166
vaginismus, 35, 169–170
Viagra, 56, 304, 309
vibrators, 209–233; addiction
to, 225; air-suction,
214; app-controlled,
229–230; apps, 222; to
boost arousal, 69–70; for
clit-owners with decreased
sensitivity, 79; clitoral,
217–218; considerations

when choosing, 219–220;
desensitization by, 224–225;
dislike of, 224; dual-action,
219; everyday objects as, 222;
first orgasms and, 53, 214;
during foreplay, 156; health
benefits, 210; history of,
211–212; kinds of, 217–221;
masturbation, 102; overview,
209–211; partnered sex,
85, 226–227; pointers for
using, 221–224; purchasing,
214–217; "rotating
unbalance" concept, 213;
as substitute for partner,
232–233; vaginal/G-spot,
218
victim, use of term, 9
video sex, 107–108
virginity, 96, 180–187
vocalizing, 259, 294, 297
vulva: anatomy/appearance
of, 60–61, 118; befriending
yours, 60–64; euphemisms
for, 24–25; photos of, 64; of
porn stars, 62–63; taste and
smell, 116–117, 120–121, 132;
use of term, 11, 23; vibrator
use on, 221, 223
vulva-owners: arousal, physical
signs of, 264; externalizing,
267; faking an orgasm,
264–271; first orgasm
stories, 51–53; masturbation
techniques, 99–100; multiple
orgasms, 33–34; oral sex,
109–141; sex involving two
vulvas, 281–291; tips for
partners of, 251–259
vulvodynia, 35, 169

watersports, 201
wetness, 31–32, 45, 166–167;
ejaculation/squirting
compared, 202; first orgasms
and, 70–71

yeast infection, 123, 138, 168